BARBARA PEARLMAN'S
DANCE EXERCISES

Barbara Pearlman's

Dance Exercises

BARBARA PEARLMAN

Photographs by Richard Blinkoff

DOLPHIN BOOKS
Doubleday & Company, Inc., Garden City, New York
1977

Library of Congress Cataloging in Publication Data

Pearlman, Barbara.
    Barbara Pearlman's dance exercises.

    1. Exercise. 2. Exercise for women.
I. Title. II. Title: Dance exercises.
GV481. P36 1977   646.7'5
ISBN 0-385-12665-4
Library of Congress Catalog Card Number 76–52009

To Stephen and Aaron

I should like to acknowledge with grateful appreciation the help of those who have made this book both possible and rewarding. Above all, my gratitude to my family who has always been loving, patient, and supportive. My thanks to Gloria Safier, for her confidence and determination. To Patrick Filley, my editor, who guided me with encouragement and sensitivity. Many thanks to Richard Blinkoff, and Bob Schlegel, Richard's assistant. My sincere gratitude to Judy Benford for her secretarial assistance. I should also like to thank those at Cinandre—Neill Stern, Wendy Whitelaw, and Linda Christiano. A special note of appreciation to Vida Jarrett. And lastly, to all my students and private clients who have, over the years, made teaching a most pleasurable and gratifying experience. To each of you, my sincere thanks.

Contents

BARBARA PEARLMAN'S
DANCE EXERCISES

Introducing Dance Exercises

The eight-week program outlined in this book is a graceful, pleasurable and, above all, effective approach to body conditioning. I call the method Dance Exercises because the majority of the sixty-four exercises in the program are similar to the warm-up movements practiced in a modern or jazz dance class. These are designed to tone, shape, and strengthen the body while simultaneously developing agility, coordination, and grace of movement. Naturally, it was necessary to modify and adapt the exercises to best suit the needs—and body—of the nondancer. For example, I have excluded movements that I consider too difficult for the average woman to execute, as well as those that require the use of a dancer's barre (a wooden rod attached to the wall at waist level). By quickly glancing through the program, you will notice that all sixty-four exercises are to be performed in a variety of positions on the floor. By eliminating the need for a standing support of any kind, it will be possible for you to practice these floor movements just about anywhere, providing you have adequate space.

Combined with the dance-oriented stretch warm-ups, I have also included some elementary yoga postures, as well as adaptations of yoga movements. These, like the dance-oriented warm-ups, are ideal for toning the body through the balance of contracting (tightening) and relaxing different muscle groups. A main yoga principle is that to be beautiful, the body must be graceful, and to be graceful, it must be supple and coordinated. Like dance, yoga aims to bring the body to its best possible shape and retain it, firm and healthy, throughout life. Through regular practice of this blend of movement techniques, you can heighten your body's capabilities and extend its range of potential. Within a mere few weeks, you will become more confident of your ability to move with ease and grace. You will also be able to place greater demands on your body instrument—not only while you exercise but as you move throughout the day.

In order for the program to be easy to follow and manageable for the average woman, I have divided it into eight weekly segments. Each segment includes two exercises for the following body areas: (1) Upper Body (neck, shoulders, arms, bosom), (2) Waist and Abdominals, (3) Hips and Buttocks, (4) Legs. This, however, is not to imply that the program is designed for "spot-reducing"—a word that does not exist in dance vocabulary. Although you may be concentrating on one area, you will simultaneously be toning and shaping other parts of the body as well. For instance, study the movement on page 102. While this exercise tones the inner thighs, it simultaneously strengthens the abdominals and firms the buttocks. Always try to relate a movement that emphasizes one part of the body to the body as a whole. You will find with most exercises some body areas will be moving while others remain stationary; be conscious of both aspects. Learn to sense the feel of the stretch, the way it affects muscles and lines that are being produced by the movement. Remember, too, while the beginning and ending of a movement are important, the path along the way is of even greater concern. That is just one of the differences between simply "getting through" a strenuous calisthenic drill and moving gracefully with controlled stretch movements.

When possible observe yourself as a dancer does, by working in front of a full-length mirror. This is particularly important when you are first learning an exercise, because it allows you to correct errors and make the proper adjustments immediately. Compare what you see in the mirror with the photograph(s). If an extreme position is illustrated, never strain or force the movement in order to achieve it. For instance, if the instructions require you to reach for your toes and you find that too difficult, reach for your calves instead. Perhaps you may never achieve the most advanced positions but you will, with regular practice, certainly increase your individual capabilities and develop a greater stretch. Each exercise involves different muscle groups and thus some movements will be easier to execute than others. Be patient and realistic. Your goal is not to achieve those "ideal measurements"—which don't really exist anyway—but instead, to live your life with greater fitness and contentment with your body. Your success with this program depends upon the recognition that your present shape took time to evolve and cannot be corrected overnight. Your figure flaws can and will be improved providing you exercise regularly with enthusiasm, patience, and resolve.

There are two fundamental dance concepts that should be kept in mind as you practice the movements. The first is that of being "centered." This means that you must consciously assemble your body in order to have total control *before* you begin to move. Centering yourself properly does not mean standing stiffly at attention; you can be centered from any starting position. It means being aware of your body and having it ready to move at your command. The second concept is "placement"; each segment of your body should be properly aligned in order to produce the correct visual unity. Placement can be either *static* or *dynamic*. When your body is motionless (as in the starting positions or in some of the sustaining positions), static placement is involved. When your body is moving, its placement constantly adjusts; this is called dynamic placement. Good placement is very important from the standpoint of effective functioning and visual line.

To derive maximum benefit from the program, you should devote an entire week to each segment—learning and mastering it to the best of your ability. When the exercises are performed at the right tempo (slowly) and without interruption, your daily practice time should take approximately fifteen minutes to complete. This includes the time devoted to the Limber-Ups (at the beginning), as well as the Deep Breathing exercise (at the end). Each session should commence with your choice of any three Limber-Ups which serve to get the blood circulating so that you are better able to perform the movements with ease and skill. At the end of each session, spend approximately two minutes (more if you wish) on the following Deep Breathing exercise: Lie on your back with your knees bent, feet resting on the floor. Place your hands gently over your rib cage. Inhale very slowly through your nose for as long as you can, making sure you feel your entire abdominal and chest areas filling up with air. Without straining, hold the air in for as long as possible. Then, very slowly, blow it out through your mouth (purse your lips as if to whistle) until your abdomen is completely empty. Use your abdominal muscles at the end to remove all the air from your lungs. Concentrate totally on your breathing, so your thoughts do not wander. After practicing this breathing technique for several days, you will be able to inhale and retain your breath for longer periods of time. Not only does this method of breathing serve to cleanse your blood (it increases the intake of oxygen and eliminates carbon dioxide), but it will further relax your mind and body at the end of each practice session. The Deep Breathing exercise can be done whenever you feel the need to calm your nerves or energize your body. It can be practiced while sitting at your desk, riding in a car (it actually works as a means of overcoming motion sickness), or just before a tense situation. One of my clients claims it works wonders for her when she has to confront the "horrors" of the dentist's chair. No matter what your reasons for using this method might be, remember to keep your breath even, relaxed, and rhythmic for maximum benefits.

The weekly segments are specifically designed to gradually become more difficult. This should pose no problems providing you follow the outlined program, and complete it at least once. If you discover that you're spending considerably less than fifteen minutes on a segment, chances are you're rushing through the exercises; try performing them at a slower tempo. In case you want to increase the amount of time you spend, you may repeat any or all of the exercises in the segment or review some of the movements you learned from earlier weeks.

None of the movements in the program place unnatural demands on your body. Nevertheless, it is advisable to check with your doctor before attempting any of the exercises if you've had a health problem or have been inactive for a significant length of time. If you are out of shape, at the beginning, you will have to summon up your discipline to follow the program regularly. At first, fifteen minutes might seem endless, especially if you're unaccustomed to exercising. You will find, however, the time really does go by quite rapidly (especially when you're listening to your favorite music) and because stretching feels so wonderful you will actually begin to look forward to the time you devote to your exercise regimen.

You need no other tools—no slant boards, ropes, weights, or expensive exercise equipment—simply a willing mind and body. You can exercise for yourself and by yourself and if you lack the patience to await the ultimate rewards, there's one benefit you will experience almost immediately; it will be the exhilarating pleasure of feeling more refreshed and vital from one day to the next.

Before You Begin

The first step before commencing with this program is to make an honest evaluation of your body by taking a good, long look at yourself in a full-length mirror—preferably with your clothes off. Ask yourself some basic questions in order to determine your personal figure and body goals: Are your muscles strong and supple? Do your legs or waistline need shaping? Is your energy level high? Do you move with ease? Can your body cope with tension? Are your upper arms firm? Is your back flexible or weak? These and many more questions should be posed and *truthfully* answered before you begin to exercise with the movements in this program.

It would be most deceptive to promise you overnight miracles and there are, quite frankly, figure conditions that simply cannot be changed. For instance, you cannot alter your basic bone structure, but you can remold and tone the flesh in order to improve your shape and appearance. Your legs can't be lengthened, but they can become more shapely. Overly pendulous breasts can't be reduced, yet you can strengthen your pectoral muscles and give your bosom a tighter, higher look. A woman's figure, however, can be transformed quite dramatically, simply by the redistribution of fat that takes place through regular exercising. Most women initially notice improvements in their thighs, hips, and buttocks (men, in their stomach and waistline). Many of my female clients discover that after regularly exercising for two months, they are able to wear slacks that were previously too tight to "squeeze" into.

If you're determined to make the most of what you were born with, exercising can and will improve your figure. Granted, you will have to practice the movements faithfully until they can be performed with ease, but don't allow your mistakes to discourage you in any way. The professional dancer invests many years of daily practice time before she is sufficiently prepared to appear in performance. You will be able to observe your own improvement and see evidence by adopting what I call the "exercise habit"—fifteen minutes of regular exercising (five days a week, once you've completed the eight-week program) with the graceful, stretch movements in this book.

Once You've Completed
The Eight-Week Program

Having completed the program exactly as it has been outlined, you may repeat it again and again, or you may use the sixty-four exercises in an endless variety of combinations (see the chart below). When creating your own fifteen-minute regimens, specifically designed for your individual needs, keep the following pointers in mind:

Always begin each session with your choice of three Limber-Ups and end with two minutes of the Deep Breathing exercise (described on page 8).

Avoid choosing exercises from only one area. Be sure to include at least one movement from each of the four categories. If you're devoting fifteen minutes a day, do not overload your routine with too many exercises. No more than ten is recommended. Keep in mind it is preferable to practice a few movements properly than many incorrectly.

Periodically, you might find it beneficial to return to the original eight-week program in order to review all of the exercises. It will not be necessary, however, to spend an entire week on each segment, since you will already be familiar with the exercises. Devote as much time as you personally wish.

	Upper Body	Waist and Abdominals	Hips and Buttocks	Legs
WEEK 1	3, 9	7, 14	1, 8	5, 12
WEEK 2	5, 7	3, 13	7, 13	10, 15
WEEK 3	1, 11	5, 9	4, 15	3, 8
WEEK 4	2, 15	8, 16	5, 11	6, 14

You need not worry that by returning to some of the earlier movements in the program your level of proficiency will diminish. Providing that you exercise regularly (and that's the key to your success), you will maintain your shape, tone, and stamina. Naturally, if you're temporarily ill or unable to exercise for several days, nothing drastic will happen; but try not to allow too much time to elapse between practice sessions.

Deep Breathing Exercise

PLACEMENT: Lie on your back with your knees bent, soles of the feet resting on the floor. Rest your hands gently on your rib cage.

MOVEMENT: Inhale very slowly through your nose, filling your abdominal and chest regions with air. Hold for as long as possible, then very slowly exhale, blowing the air out through your mouth until your abdomen is completely empty.

TOTAL REPETITION: Two minutes.

Helpful Hints
for More Successful Exercising

. . . Try whenever possible to exercise at the same time each day since you are less apt to forget. Thereby exercising will become part of your daily routine. Just about any time is fine, except directly after meals or right before bedtime. Since these movements have a refreshing, revitalizing effect, you should limit late night exercising to the Relaxercises.

. . . The best and most valuable time to exercise depends on your personal preference and your daily schedule. Many of my clients prefer the morning, before their day becomes busy and hectic. If, on the other hand, you're not an "early bird" or the morning hours are too frenetic, you might spend the time later in the day when you're most in need of an energy boost. Whatever time you choose, it should be when you are not harried. A successful practice session should relax your mind, as well as tone your body; substituting speed for thoroughness is not beneficial.

. . . The program's effectiveness depends upon your actual involvement in the movements. Try to focus on the stretching process as it affects the various parts of your body. By truly concentrating you can give total attention to correct technique and proper body alignment. To involve yourself and enjoy the movements as you perform them contributes not only to the physical effectiveness, but to the mental usefulness as well. If you're tense or upset when you begin, by totally concentrating on the movements and your breathing, you will revive your body and relieve your mind of problems. When the fifteen minutes are up, you'll feel amazingly refreshed.

. . . Make certain the room is well ventilated and free of drafts, since muscles tend to cramp when they're cold. Should you be unable to exercise on a carpet, and object to a bare floor, use a towel, scatter rug, or exercise mat—if you have one.

. . . The best attire for exercising is one that permits maximum freedom of movement. A leotard and tights (in which every bulge is obvious)

9

is the actual practice clothing a dancer wears. This attire keeps your muscles warm because of its clinging nature, and allows you to actually see the various parts of your body stretching. If you do not choose to wear a leotard and tights (most of my male clients do not), make certain your clothing does not inhibit movement in any way.

. . . Avoid resting in between exercises for more than a few seconds. Stopping for extended periods is not only time-consuming, but will cause you to lose the sustaining effects of the movements. You will also find it more difficult to resume if you break your rhythm.

. . . Don't push yourself beyond capacity. If you do, especially if you've been inactive, you'll become discouraged and lose interest. Take it slowly at first. If the instructions call for repeating the movement sixteen times and you find that too demanding, build up to it gradually. If you are really out of shape, the fifteen minutes might have to be somewhat reduced at first; let your body be your guide. In the beginning, since your muscles are being used in unaccustomed ways, you might experience some muscle soreness. Lazy muscles, inactive for a considerable amount of time, are naturally going to protest; this is absolutely normal and should not cause any concern. Muscle discomfort can best be treated by simply repeating the same kind of movements. Soaking in a warm bath also helps to ease soreness. As the days progress, providing you're regular about exercising, you will notice that the minor aches you formerly experienced disappear. So don't allow a bit of initial discomfort to prevent you from continuing with the program.

. . . I wouldn't consider exercising without music. In a dance class, there is always some kind of accompaniment—records, a piano, or the beat of drums. Music not only helps you execute movements with greater rhythm and grace, but it adds considerably to the enjoyment of your practice time. The music need not be a steady four-four beat. You might prefer the Beatles one day and Beethoven the next. I use a variety of music —calypso, jazz, folk, or even the scores from favorite Broadway shows—it depends on my mood. Select music that appeals to you; that's all that really counts.

. . . At the beginning of each of the eight weeks, in order to perform the exercises correctly, I suggest you do the following: First, study the photograph(s) which will give you a general impression of the exercise. Then read the accompanying instructions slowly, just as you would study a detailed recipe. (Make certain to read the check notes as well.) Then reread the instructions for each exercise as you slowly pace through the movement. As soon as you fully comprehend the entire segment, you're ready to begin. Remember, unless indicated in the instructions, all the movements should be done slowly and evenly.

Proper Breathing While You Exercise

The manner in which you breathe while exercising directly affects the nature of the movements of your body—both internally and externally. When many of my clients first begin to exercise, the tendency is to hold their breath because they are placing total emphasis and concentration on performing the movements correctly. Yet, it is most important that you avoid holding your breath, because it robs you of energy and lessens your ability to move with strength and ease.

The simplest manner to describe the recommended breathing technique for exercising is the following: Inhale when you need maximum strength for the movement and exhale when your body is releasing or relaxing. Any lifted movement, when accompanied by an inhalation of breath, will become fuller and more enriched. By way of illustration, center your body in a standing position and rise to the balls of your feet (in ballet this is called a relevé). Simultaneously lift your arms upward and inhale deeply. Now, repeat the same motion, but this time, exhale while you lift your arms and body. Were you aware of how the two different ways of breathing affected the movement? You probably found you were able to lift with greater ease while inhaling.

Breathing gives important support to the dancer's movements. She learns to control it and become aware of how to use it to her advantage. During a contraction or when a movement is drawn inward, the breath should always be expelled. You will thus discover that you will generally inhale when you stretch, reach, lift, or raise your body and exhale when you bend or bring your limbs close to your body. The following movement should illustrate this point: Stand with your feet slightly apart. Take a deep breath through your nose and begin to lift both arms upward. Hold the position for several counts, then exhale, letting your back round and your arms and head dangle limply. Maintain the released position for several counts before you begin to slowly inhale and uncurl the body to a straight-back position. With each new movement that you learn, try to be conscious of the correct breathing process that will be most effective for the particular exercise. This will allow you to execute the movement with maximum strength and skill.

The Importance of Regular Exercise

It is unfortunate but true that most people do not derive sufficient exercise during the course of a day to keep their bodies attractive and healthy. We drive short distances in lieu of walking, and use elevators and escalators instead of climbing stairs. We even spare ourselves the simple motions of sharpening a pencil, opening a can, or brushing our teeth. Mechanical devices in this "push-button age" have diminished or totally eliminated the need for muscular effort. What ensues, unfortunately, from prolonged inactivity is a state of muscle deterioration and overall body weakness. Consider the effects that extended bed rest have on a normal person and you will, undoubtedly, understand the importance of regular exercise. Inactivity not only results in the loss of muscle tone and elasticity, but causes stiffness of the joints, slowed-down circulation, glandular lethargy, and the accumulation of fats and toxins. Even the complexion suffers. Many of these conditions are generally associated with "old age," yet they can, and do, occur in people of all ages.

When you exercise regularly, even your sex life is affected and enhanced. Your mental outlook is bound to be more positive if you look and feel your best. You will have additional confidence and self-esteem when you're pleased and proud of the way you look. Feeling good about yourself in turn heightens your potential for giving as well as receiving. If you feel good about yourself you are apt to be freer, more natural and spontaneous with your lover. A body that moves with grace, ease, and assurance is a more exciting, sensual one.

You will discover, as you become familiar with the movements in this program, that many are specifically designed to strengthen the back and abdominal muscles, as well as develop gluteal (seat) and pelvic control—all important for pleasurable lovemaking. By developing command over your body, a fuller, happier, more satisfying sex life will be enjoyed.

Men and the Dance Exercise Program

In writing this book I have frequently alluded to the female anatomy, which should not, however, imply that men cannot also benefit from the movements in this program. This system of exercise designed to tone, strengthen, energize, and proportion the body will be just as effective for trimming and shaping a man's physique. A man who actively participates in sports certainly recognizes the need for flexibility and muscle tone. Accidents, on the ski slopes or tennis courts, generally occur when one's muscles and joints are insufficiently prepared for movement. My husband makes it a point to exercise with these stretch movements daily and is truly convinced that they are an ideal preparation for the rigors of his early morning tennis game.

One of my clients, a vice-president of a large corporation, works in what he describes as a "pressure cooker" environment. Two years ago, he organized a group of men for a weekly lunchtime "stretch session" in his office. They all agree that exercising helps them cope with the frustrations of an average business day. My guess is these sessions relax them far more than that all-too-popular businessman's martini—and think of the calories they save.

Another client, a writer, began lessons several years ago in order to increase his energy and stamina. He was generally feeling lethargic and fatigued, largely due to a daily life almost totally devoid of physical activity. He remained faithful to his lessons (and regular practice sessions) and has made significant progress. His endurance has improved considerably, as well as his postural habits. Whenever he feels tired or tense, as a result of extended periods at the typewriter, he pushes his chair away from his desk and takes time out for a few minutes of refreshing stretch movements.

Some of my female clients exercise at a time that is equally convenient for their husbands; many couples discover stretching together can be quite pleasurable. One couple, both free-lance writers working at home, exercise regularly at about four in the afternoon—just when they feel the need for an energizing lift. If you exercise with the man in your life, try to encourage him to follow a regular regimen. Not only will you be pleased with his appearance, but, more importantly, he will gain increased vitality that will insure him of a fuller, more satisfying life.

Weight Control and Exercise

No exercise program can, or should, guarantee weight reduction. Losing pounds can only happen by changing your eating habits and accepting the fact that, unfortunately, calories do count. A calorie represents a specific amount of energy in the form of heat, created by your body's burning up of a specific amount of food. Fat accumulates (on the hips, buttocks, upper arms, etc.) when you consume more calories than you are able to burn up in daily activity. Naturally, the more active you are, the more calories you are able to consume. That is one reason it is so important to limit your late night eating or snacking, if you want to lose weight; there's simply no time to adequately burn up those calories.

Many women I meet express the fact that they are careful about their diets but nevertheless are unable to lose weight. I suggest you do the following for an entire week: Keep a record (and it will take time and effort) of everything you eat, and all beverages you consume. It is not necessary, however, to note *exact* quantities. Use index cards or a small pad so that you can carry your notes in your purse during the day. At the end of the week, examine the list carefully and critically. Chances are you'll be quite amazed (as so many of my clients are) how many "cheats" you indulged in. For so many women, simply seeing the facts in writing helps to increase their discipline and determination to lose those extra pounds.

Neglecting to exercise while you diet is not advisable. Although you might become thinner, your skin will sag and lack tone and you will look years older than you actually are. Besides, a weight-reduction program lacking stimulating physical activity can become boring and tedious. The facts are quite simple: Diet decreases pounds; exercise shapes and streamlines the figure. The two should go hand in hand. Through regular exercising, you will also develop greater confidence and awareness of your body—not only while practicing the various movements, but as you move throughout the day. Since these movements serve to relax the mind and body, you won't eat as much during periods of tension. When you have the urge for a high-calorie snack, take the time it would require to prepare (and eat) it and spend the time exercising, instead. Or, you might simply choose to practice the Deep Breathing exercise. Most of the time, you'll discover the craving will diminish considerably or entirely pass. Begin to substitute action thoughts for food thoughts and you'll be on the right road to weight reduction and figure control.

The Five Major Areas

NECK AND SHOULDERS

Two areas which are apt to be most affected by tension are the shoulders and the back of the neck. You will find that taking time out for simple stretch movements, when you feel tense or fatigued, can often prevent painful spasms from developing. These easy exercises take little time, are quite inconspicuous, and will certainly help to loosen muscles that tend to tighten quite unconsciously. Slowly lifting and lowering the shoulders (shrugs) or forming slow circular motions (rotations) can be effective for relieving strain. So too is the head roll when done smoothly and slowly. If you close your eyes and try to relax as you gently roll your head in a circular motion, you will almost immediately feel the tension lessening.

Many people, due to the nature of their jobs, round their shoulders so habitually that they remain hunched permanently. This causes the pectoral muscles to foreshorten and places constant stress on the back muscles, which eventually lose their strength and elasticity. Strengthening the pectoral and upper back muscles can help to correct a round-shouldered condition. Many of the Upper Body movements throughout this program (especially those in which the hands are clasped behind the body and the arms are slowly lifted) are particularly effective for correcting this postural problem.

Sitting at a desk for endless hours with your head down can cause the nerves of the neck to become taut and rigid. As a result, you're apt to develop either a "tension headache" or a "stiff neck"—sometimes both. No matter how busy you might be, it's essential that you occasionally lift your head and chest and relax your shoulders. Try this exercise occasionally while sitting at your desk: Simply inhale deeply as you simultaneously raise your arms overhead. Stretch as high as you can. Feel your torso separating from your hip area, then relax. (Taking time out for a minute or

18

two of stretching at intervals during your work day can serve to refresh and clear your mind, and thus enhance your productivity.) Or, try this helpful neck-relaxing exercise when you arrive home at the end of a hectic, tension-filled day: Lie on your bed with your knees bent and your arms resting at your sides. Hang your head over the edge of the bed, being certain that your neck is fully supported. Close your eyes and just let your head hang for a minute or two. Then slowly roll it from side to side. This movement not only relieves neck strain, but strengthens the jaw muscles as well.

Try not to tighten or tense your shoulders as you practice the various movements in this program. By holding them in a rigid manner, you are placing unnecessary stress on the chest muscles. This causes the entire body to be pulled out of line. Also be conscious of stretching your neck as long and as gracefully as possible—like that of a dancer. Although some exercises do require you to contract your neck muscles (for example, in order to support your head as you lift it off of the floor), generally, the neck should be held loose and relaxed.

ARMS AND BOSOM

A woman is generally unaware of her upper arms until that dreadful moment when she discovers they've become loose and flabby. If you've neglected to exercise regularly, chances are your upper arms (the underneath portion in particular) need firming and toning. You need not worry that by exercising you will acquire bulgy arm muscles. The slow, nonstrenuous stretch movements in this program will develop tone in the arm muscles, which consequently means tighter, more attractive skin. If you're familiar with the backstroke in swimming (which is marvelous exercise for the upper arms), you can do the same movement out of the water with approximately the same results. Start by moving one arm up and then back in a big circle. As the arm reaches the top of the circle, begin the same motion with your other arm. This not only shapes the upper arms, but tightens the bosom as well.

Arm Rotation Movement

PLACEMENT: Stand with your feet comfortably apart, arms resting at your sides.

MOVEMENT: Begin by lifting the right arm up and then behind in a big circle. As the arm reaches the top of the circle, start the same motion with the left arm. Keep the movement steady and avoid halting at any point.

TOTAL REPETITION: Twelve times.

Since the breasts are chiefly fatty tissue, it would be deceptive to state that exercising can drastically change the appearance of the bosom. The breasts will not become larger or smaller from exercise. What exercising can do is strengthen the muscles of the chest and shoulders which support the breasts. By toning the pectoral muscles, you can give your bosom a higher, tighter appearance.

Remember, too, correct posture is absolutely esstential for the beauty of the bustline. A round-shouldered carriage will naturally cause the bosom to sag and droop. Try to be cognizant of correct body alignment as you sit, stand, and move about.

WAIST AND ABDOMINALS

Although I have grouped the waist and abdominals together in the course of the program, they are not to be confused. It is possible to have a small waistline but a flaccid, toneless belly. Generally, however, this is not the case, since weak abdominals usually indicate poor overall body tone. Lack of abdominal tone also throws the body out of line. When the abdominal muscles are weak, the back invariably suffers, since the abdominals are the chief means of frontal support for the spine.

Fundamental to all dance techniques are tilting, bending, twisting motions, all so effective for trimming and toning the waist and abdominal areas. In the check notes for many of the Waist and Abdominal movements, you will be reminded to *keep your buttocks stationary* as you stretch to the side. With the buttocks firmly placed (see page 95), you are actually creating a resisting force which allows for a more effective stretch. In movements where an overhead stretching motion is indicated (see page 51), try to hold your rib cage as high as possible, thus separating it from the hip area. By doing so, you will again be maximizing the stretch through the torso area.

It is most important to strengthen your natural girdle of muscle if the muscles in your midsection are weak. One effective toning exercise can be done while sitting, standing, or even lying down: Pull your abdominals in and try to maintain the contraction for about eight slow counts. Be certain, however, that you do not hold your breath. Repeat this simple isometric exercise whenever you can remember—while on the telephone, in the tub, or preparing dinner for your family. The more frequently you practice it, the better control you will have of your muscles. Also try to use every opportunity throughout the day to reach, twist, bend, and stretch. This not only trims the waistline, but keeps your body agile and supple.

In the mornings, I frequently do the following stretch before getting out of bed. I also recommend it if you're temporarily bedridden, since it helps prevent stiffness from developing: Lying flat, extend your legs in front and your arms overhead. Rest your hands on the bed with your palms facing upward. Alternating sides, *very* slowly stretch overhead with the right arm (as far as possible), then with the left. Repeat this stretch for a minute or two. Not only does it feel quite marvelous (especially in the morning, when you're somewhat stiff), but it tones and tightens the waistline as well.

HIPS AND BUTTOCKS

For many of my female clients (especially those over forty with sedentary jobs), the hips and buttocks seem to be the most problematic areas. Generally, large buttocks and oversized hips are a combined problem. In many cases, a weight-reduction diet coupled with exercising regularly is necessary. Women whose work keeps them active and on the move are much less apt to have problems with large hips and buttocks than those who sit a great deal of the day.

How you sit can also make a difference (this applies to the manner in which you sit while exercising as well). Most women tend to sit with their bodies improperly placed. Instead of sitting slightly forward in a chair, they sit back on the largest part of their buttocks and thus encourage further spreading. It's not simply a matter of keeping the back erect, but of leaning slightly forward so that the weight is shifted from the hips. For example, when you're talking on the telephone, instead of slouching back in your chair, lean forward and shift the placement of your weight. This subtle adjustment can really make a difference.

It is most important, if you're relatively inactive all day, that you make an additional effort to get as much exercise as possible during nonworking hours. This is not only essential for the shape of your figure, but for your overall health and well-being. Are you accustomed to driving everywhere, even short distances? Then try walking or riding a bike, instead. Walk to work if you possibly can. Give up your seat on the bus or subway and stand. Just balancing yourself (by contracting the buttock muscles) is a good form of exercise. When you do walk, take deep breaths and long, rapid strides—don't just stroll casually. Also make an effort to supplement your regular exercise regimen with an invigorating, stimulating sport that appeals to you.

Although most women have "given up the girdle," there are still many who rely on it to keep them held together. However, wearing a girdle daily is not advisable, since it restricts the flow of blood to the lower parts of the body. It also holds up lazy muscles, preventing them from developing support of their own. Think of it this way: Imagine that every time you wanted to lift your leg, someone lifted it for you. In time, the muscles would lose their elasticity and eventually atrophy. Wearing a girdle presents a similar situation, eventually the buttock muscles become weak and simply give up.

In a dance class, one often hears the instructor reminding a pupil to "tuck the buttocks under." This is done by contracting the gluteal (seat) muscles and pushing the pelvis slightly forward. Practice and perfect the "buttock tuck" in profile in front of a full-length mirror. Then, once you've mastered it, you can do it just about anywhere because of its invisible nature. Never frown on taking time for these extra "sneaky" exercises. Use every possible opportunity to make your muscles work for you. The more you use them, the better use you'll get from them, which in turn means a fitter, more attractive you.

Isometric Buttock Tuck

PLACEMENT: Stand with your feet wide apart and parallel, hands resting on your waist.

MOVEMENT: Grip the buttocks in a tight contraction, pushing the pelvis slightly forward. Hold for six slow counts, then release.

TOTAL REPETITION: Eight times.

THE LEG

The entire leg, from the thigh to the foot, requires regular exercise in order to remain strong and attractive. The shape of the thighs, calves, and ankles, as well as the strength of the knees and feet, can be enhanced through regular practice of the stretch movements in this program. Should your thighs be excessively heavy, you might have to combine massage (to break up thick tissue where fat is trapped) with your exercise regimen. Try to avoid crossing your legs while sitting; this only further thickens the thighs by cutting down on vital circulation. Shift positions whenever possible if you sit for extended periods of time. By doing so, you will prevent the tissues in the thighs from constantly being compressed.

Place particular emphasis on all the leg-bending movements in the program if your knees are weak and stiff. Also begin each day's practice session with the plié (page 31), which has been included as one of the Limber-Ups. This movement is basic to all dance techniques and should be practiced slowly and evenly. Keep your back straight and your buttocks "tucked under" as you bend your knees. You might do some pliés as soon as you get out of bed in the morning if your legs feel particularly rigid. Also try to walk as much as you possibly can in order to tone the legs and strengthen the knees.

Calves, be they straight as sticks or somewhat too heavy (which is more difficult to correct), can be partially improved with exercise. Walking barefoot, high on the balls of your feet, is an effective way to develop your calf muscles. Make a conscious effort to point your feet while practicing the movements in this program, if your calves lack contour. On the other hand, if they are large and somewhat bulgy, avoid pointing your feet excessively. Flex them instead. Flexing (the opposite of pointing) is when the toes are pulled back. toward your leg and the heel is pressed downward.

Even the most attractive, slender legs can be marred by fat, swollen ankles. In some cases, heaviness is due to actual bone structure, but more often it results from the accumulation of fat and the lack of exercise. One way to slim and strengthen the ankle is to practice the foot rotation movement. This exercise can be done while sitting in a chair as well. Just lift your foot slightly off the floor and rotate it in a clockwise direction several times, then in a counterclockwise direction. It's possible that you might hear some strange snapping, cracking sounds. Don't worry, it's simply stiffness which will subside once the joints in the ankle and foot become looser. I suggest that my clients practice the foot rotation exercise during long plane flights in order to prevent ankle swelling and stiffness.

Try, for your feet's sake, to walk as much as you possibly can. You don't have to run or jog, simply walk. The chief way that blood comes up from the lower extremities is by action of the muscles on the veins. Naturally, your circulation will be affected if the muscles lack exercise. Since the feet are so far away from the heart, circulation has to be consistently worked on. Massaging the feet also helps your circulation and combats tiredness as well. Or, try wiggling your toes in your shoes once in a while when your feet begin to get stiff during the day. You might also put your feet up occasionally, not just off the floor but higher than your heart. This improves your circulation by easing the flow through your legs and down to your feet.

The Eight-Week Dance Exercise Program

Limber-Ups (1)

PLACEMENT: Stand with your feet apart and parallel. Clasp your hands behind your body, arms straight.

MOVEMENT: Round the back and drop the head as you simultaneously lift the arms. In this position, bounce up and down five times. Pull the arms back into place as you slowly straighten the body to the original position.

TOTAL REPETITION: Ten times.

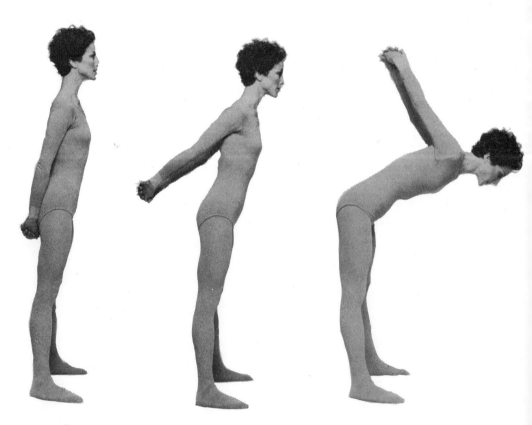

Limber-Ups (2)

PLACEMENT: Stand with your feet wide apart and slightly turned out. Extend your arms overhead, palms facing in.

MOVEMENT: In an even, tilting motion, stretch the arms and torso from side to side six times. Relax for three slow counts, then repeat.

TOTAL REPETITION: Three times.

Try to keep the head and neck as relaxed as possible as you tilt from side to side.

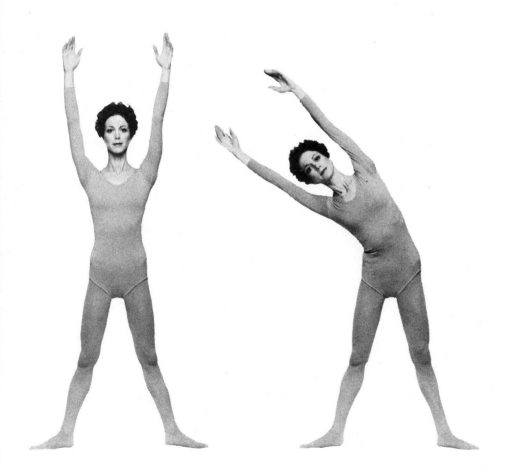

Limber-Ups (3)

PLACEMENT: Stand with feet wide apart and parallel, hands resting on the waist.

MOVEMENT: Release the torso forward, keeping the shoulders pulled back and the head slightly lifted. In this flat back position, bounce gently up and down two times. Round the shoulders, drop the head, and uncurl the body to the original position. Take two counts for each part of this torso roll.

TOTAL REPETITION: Ten times.

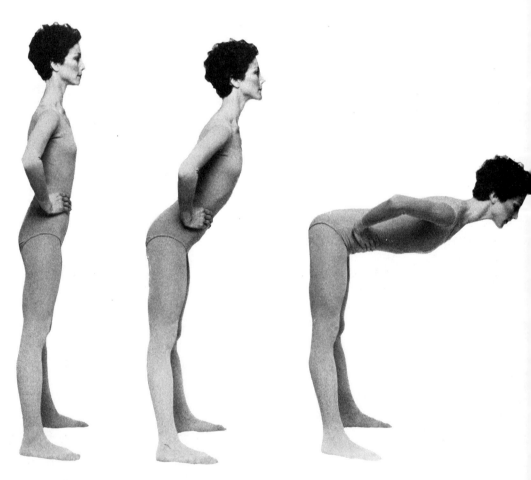

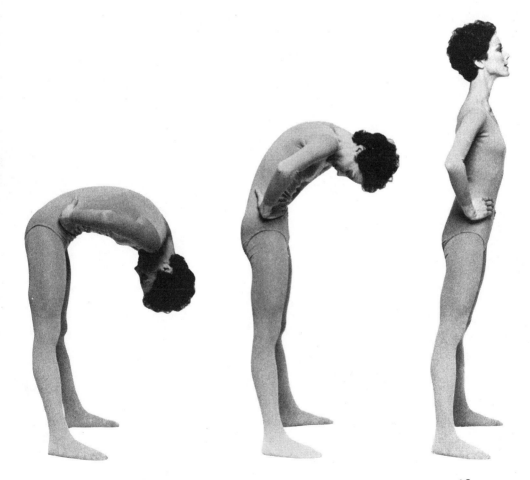

Limber-Ups (4)

PLACEMENT: Stand with your feet about twelve inches apart and parallel, arms relaxed at your sides.

MOVEMENT: Round your back, lower your head, and release your body over the right leg. Clasp your hands around the ankle (or the calf if it is more comfortable) and gently bounce up and down four times. Pull your head as close to your leg as you can. Repeat on the left leg. Then repeat with your hands clasped around both ankles. Uncurl the body slowly to the original position.

TOTAL REPETITION: Three times.

This exercise not only strengthens the hamstring muscles but firms the buttocks as well.

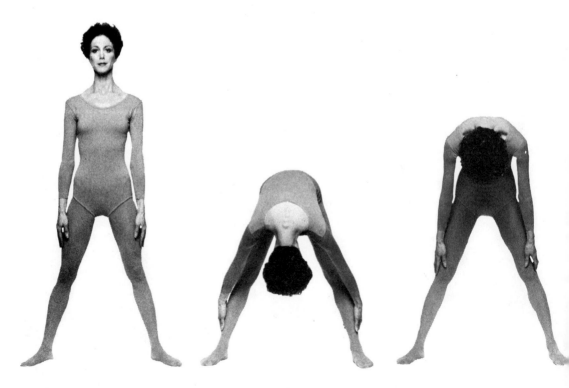

Limber-Ups (5)

PLACEMENT: Stand with your feet wide apart and slightly turned out. Rest your hands on your waist. Hold your back erect.

MOVEMENT: Bend the knees, keeping the soles of the feet on the floor and the buttocks tucked under. Bounce up and down four times without straightening the legs. Keep the shoulders pulled back. Resume original position.

TOTAL REPETITION: Eight times.

The plié can also be done by slowly bending then straightening the legs—without the bounce. Try it both ways.

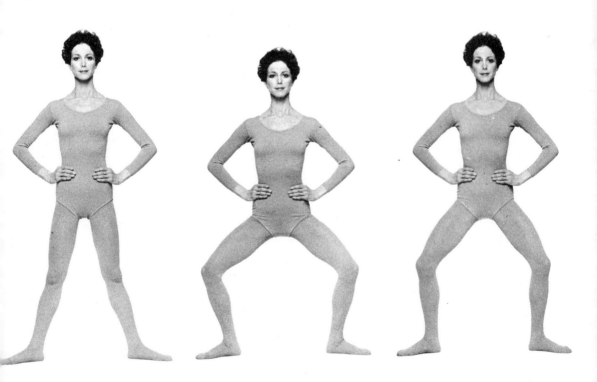

FIRST WEEK

Upper Body (1)

PLACEMENT: Sit with the ankles crossed, back held erect. Clasp your hands behind your head, elbows open to the sides.

MOVEMENT: Slowly bring the elbows together. Open the elbows to resume the original position.

TOTAL REPETITION: Twelve times.

Exhale as the elbows come together, inhale as they open to the sides.

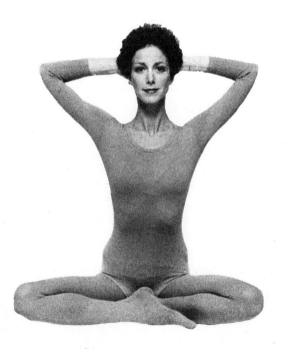
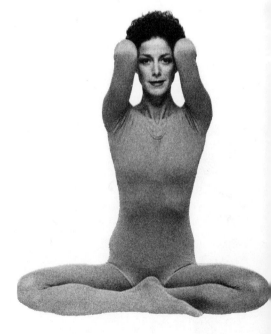

Upper Body (2)

PLACEMENT: Lie on floor with legs extended in front, toes pointed, arms relaxed at your sides.

MOVEMENT: Lift head, neck, and shoulders off the floor. Hold for two counts and release. Repeat four times, then slowly roll the head from side to side four times.

TOTAL REPETITION: Three times.

Whenever lifting the head off the floor, drop the chin forward so that you do not place unnecessary stress on the neck muscles.

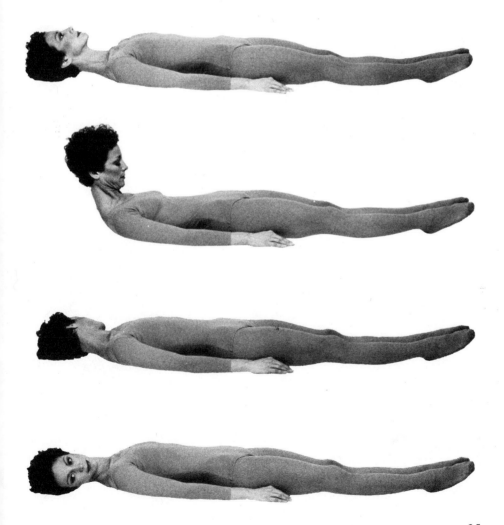

Waist and Abdominals (1)

PLACEMENT: Sit with ankles crossed, hands resting on the knees.

MOVEMENT: Lean to the right and begin a swiveling, circular movement with the torso (right, forward, left, center). Repeat the motion four times, reverse direction and do the same to the left.

TOTAL REPETITION: Two times to each side.

As you rotate the body, try to lean as far to each side and as close to the floor as you can. Do not allow the shoulders to stiffen, let them move naturally with the motion of the torso. Keep the buttocks flat on the floor as the body rotates.

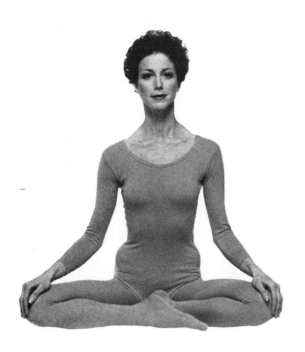

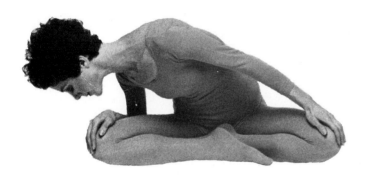

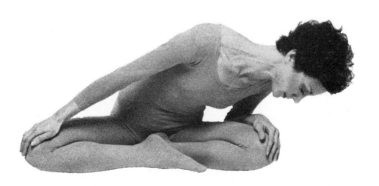

Waist and Abdominals (2)

PLACEMENT: Sit with your legs extended in front, feet together, toes pointed, back held erect. Raise the arms overhead, palms facing in.

MOVEMENT: Drop the head, round the back, and reach for your toes. Hold this position for two counts, then lift the body and arms to the original position.

TOTAL REPETITION: Ten times.

In order to derive a greater stretch for the back of the legs, you can do this same movement with your feet in a flexed position.

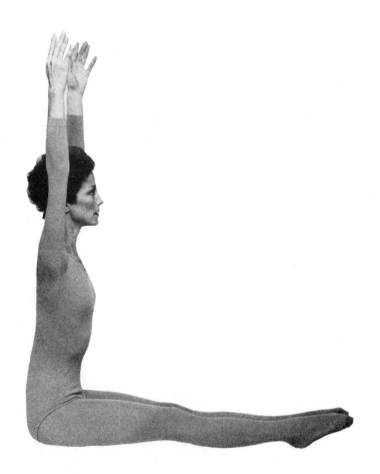

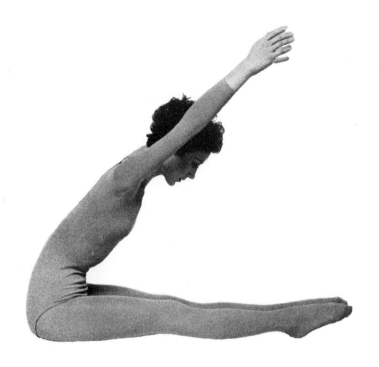

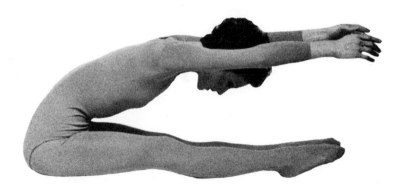

Hips and Buttocks (1)

PLACEMENT: Sit with ankles crossed, hands resting on the knees.

MOVEMENT: Twist the body from the waist, trying to touch your left cheek to your right knee. Look over your right shoulder and gently bounce up and down four times. Return center and repeat to the left.

TOTAL REPETITION: Four times to each side.

Try to keep your abdominals contracted and your buttocks flat on the floor throughout this movement.

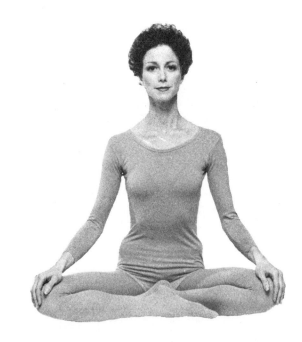

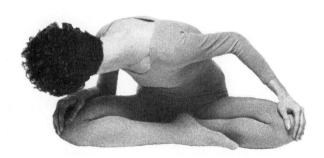

Hips and Buttocks (2)

PLACEMENT: Lie on the floor with your legs extended in front, toes pointed. The arms should be stretched overhead on the floor with the palms facing up.

MOVEMENT: Contract the buttock muscles tightly and hold for three slow counts. Draw your knees to your chest as you lower your arms to the floor at your sides, palms facing down; hold this position for three counts.

TOTAL REPETITION: Eight times.

The buttock contraction is an isometric exercise for toning and developing control of the buttock muscles. You can do this contraction while standing or sitting as well.

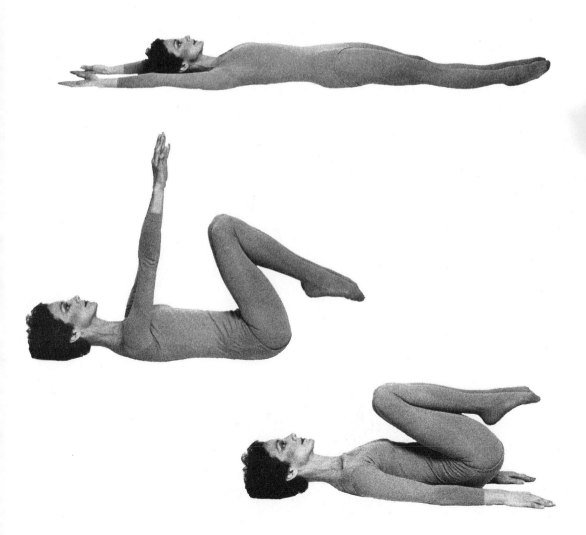

Legs (1)

PLACEMENT: Lie on the floor, hands on the hips. Extend the legs in front, toes pointed.

MOVEMENT: Bend the right leg, drawing the knee close to the chest. Extend the leg upward until it is straight. Release the leg to the floor. Repeat ten times, then repeat on the left leg.

TOTAL REPETITION: Two times on each leg.

As you release the leg to the floor, keep your abdominals contracted and press your spine into the floor so that it remains flat.

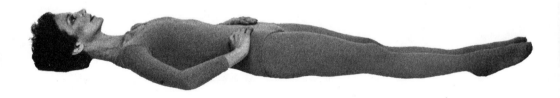

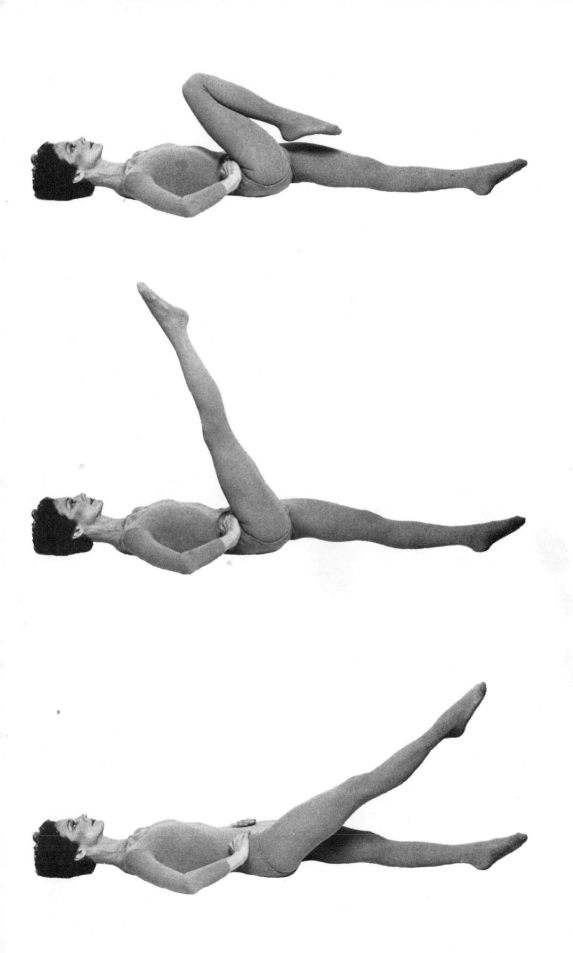

Legs (2)

PLACEMENT: Lie on the floor with the left leg extended in front and the foot turned out. Bend the right leg, rest the foot on top of the left thigh. Hands rest on your waist.

MOVEMENT: In a quick, rhythmic motion, bounce the right knee up and down sixteen times. Repeat on the left leg.

TOTAL REPETITION: Three times on each leg.

Try to lower the knee as close to the floor without lifting the opposite buttock. This is an excellent toner for the inner thigh.

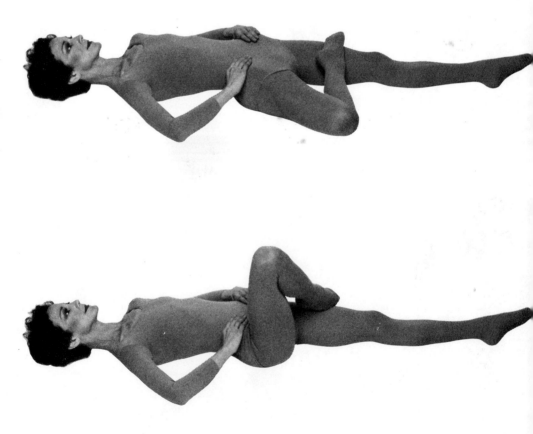

SECOND WEEK

Upper Body (3)

PLACEMENT: Sit with the legs extended in front, toes pointed, hands clasped behind the head, elbows open to the sides.

MOVEMENT: Round the back, lower the head, and bring the elbows together. Hold for three counts before lifting the body and opening the elbows to the original position.

TOTAL REPETITION: Twelve times.

This exercise is particularly beneficial for correcting round shoulders.

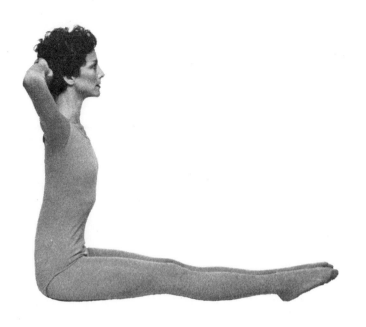

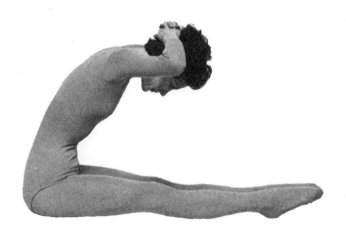

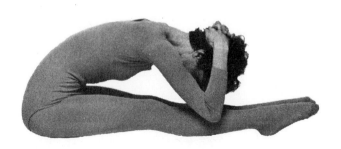

47

Upper Body (4)

PLACEMENT: Sit with the ankles crossed, back held erect. Clasp your hands behind your body, keeping the arms straight.

MOVEMENT: Slowly, lift and lower the arms without moving the upper body.

TOTAL REPETITION: Twelve times.

As your arms become more flexible, you will find it easier to raise them. Take it slowly at first and do not force this movement. This exercise is very effective for strengthening the pectoral muscles.

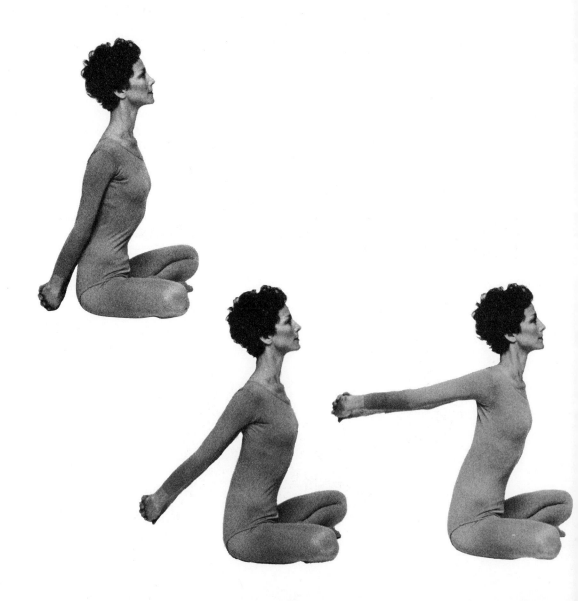

Waist and Abdominals (3)

PLACEMENT: Lie on the floor with your knees bent, feet parallel and about ten inches apart. Relax your arms at your sides.

MOVEMENT: Press your spine against the floor by contracting your abdominal muscles and hold for three counts. Slowly lift your head, neck, shoulders, and arms off the floor. Hold this position for three counts before releasing to the original position.

TOTAL REPETITION: Eight times.

As you lift your head off the floor, make certain to drop the chin forward. There will normally be some tightening of the neck muscles in order to support the head as it lifts off the floor.

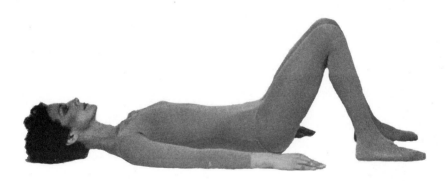

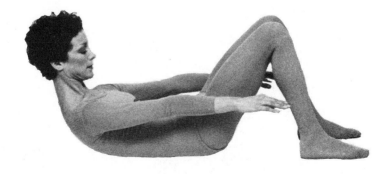

Waist and Abdominals (4)

PLACEMENT: Sit with your ankles crossed, hands resting at your sides on the floor.

MOVEMENT: Lean your body as far right as possible. At the same time, slide the right arm away from the body as the left arm arches overhead with the palm facing up. Repeat the stretch to the left.

TOTAL REPETITION: Ten times to each side.

This movement should be performed slowly for maximum effectiveness. It is important that the buttocks remain stationary as the body stretches sideways. As you lean to the right, resist by pressing the left buttock down. Do the same to the left.

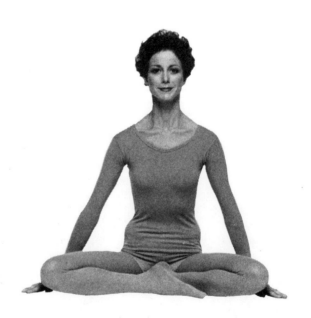

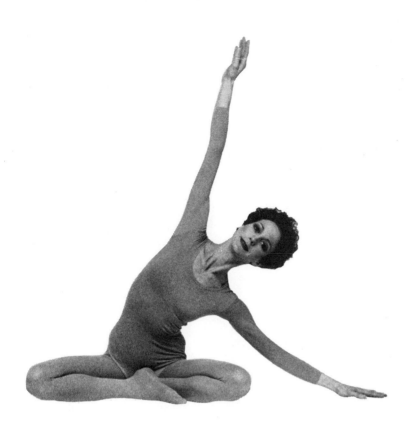

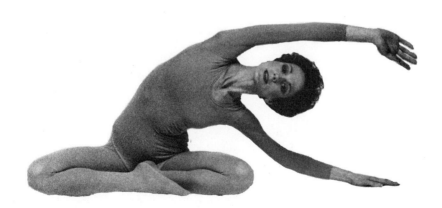

Hips and Buttocks (3)

PLACEMENT: Lie on your back with your knees drawn close to your chest. Rest your hands on your waist.

MOVEMENT: Keeping the knees together throughout this movement, rotate them in a full circle to the right four times, then to the left.

TOTAL REPETITION: Two times to each side.

Try to roll the knees as far to each side as possible without lifting the shoulders off the floor. As the knees release away from the body, the back will arch slightly. As they draw close to the chest the spine should flatten against the floor.

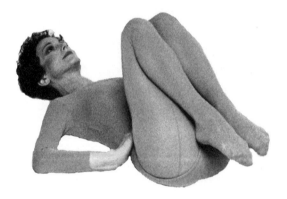

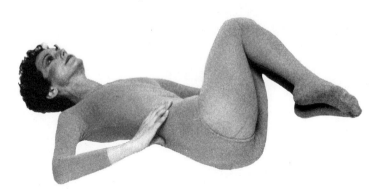

Hips and Buttocks (4)

PLACEMENT: Lie on your back, legs extended in front, toes pointed, heels touching, feet turned out. Rest your hands on your hips.

MOVEMENT: Swing the right leg as far to the side as possible. It need not raise more than several inches off the floor. Swing it back into place. Repeat six times, then repeat on the left leg.

TOTAL REPETITION: Three times on each leg.

It is important to keep the foot of the leg that is not swinging turned out. By doing so, you will prevent the buttock from lifting off the floor. This exercise is also very effective for toning the inner thigh.

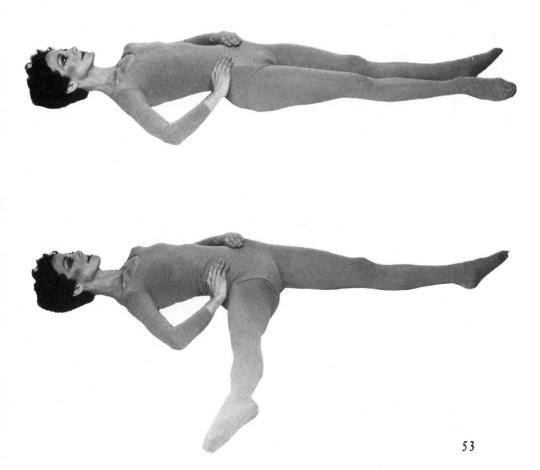

Legs (3)

PLACEMENT: Lie on your back with your knees drawn close to your chest. Arms rest at your sides.

MOVEMENT: Extend both legs upward until they are straight, then bend them to the original position. Repeat four times. Draw the knees close to your chest with your hands and rock forward and back with the knees four times.

TOTAL REPETITION: Five times.

This leg extension is also very effective for strengthening the abdominal muscles.

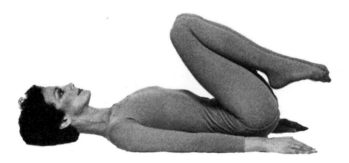

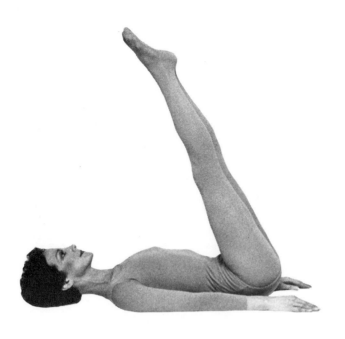

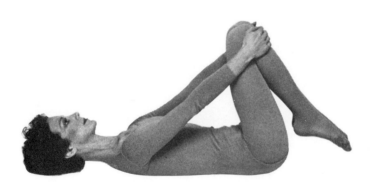

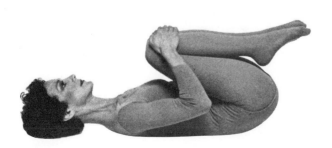

Legs (4)

PLACEMENT: Lie on your back. Bend the left leg and rest the foot on the floor. The right leg is extended upward. Hands rest on your waist.

MOVEMENT: Slowly rotate the right foot from the ankle in an outward direction six times. Next, point and flex the foot six times. Repeat on the left foot.

TOTAL REPETITION: Two times on each foot.

Rotating and flexing the foot not only strengthens the ankles but enhances the circulation of the foot as well.

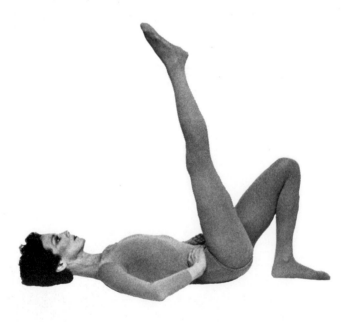

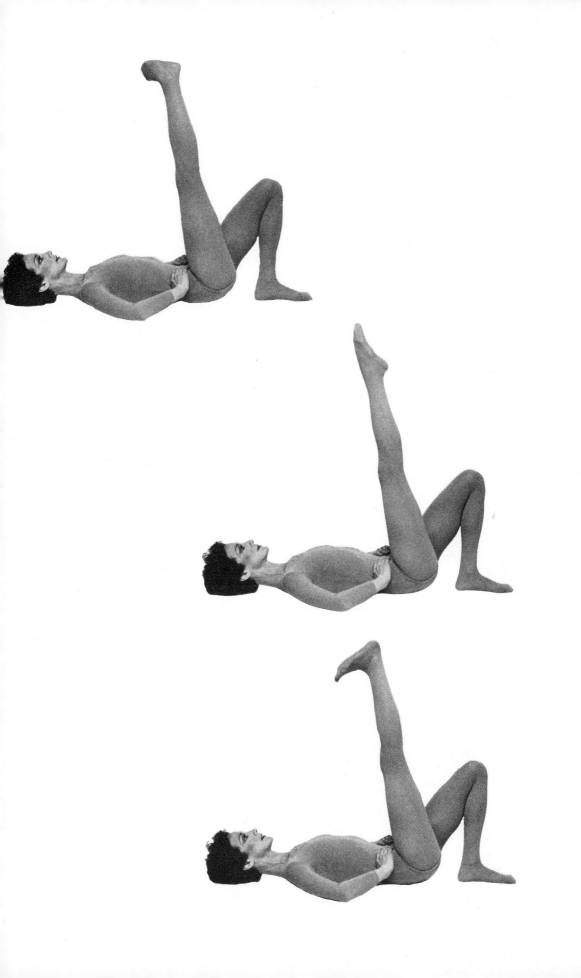

THIRD WEEK

Upper Body (5)

PLACEMENT: Sit with your ankles crossed, hands resting on your knees.

MOVEMENT: Release your body forward from the waist, pulling the shoulders back and keeping the back from rounding. Then drop your head, round your shoulders, and contract your abdominal muscles. Finally, beginning from the lower spine, uncurl your body to the original position. Take two slow counts for each part of this movement.

TOTAL REPETITION: Eight times.

Try to do this torso roll in a rhythmic, fluid motion without halting at any point. Remember to exhale as you release forward and inhale as you uncurl.

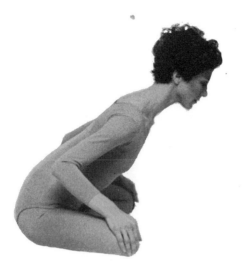

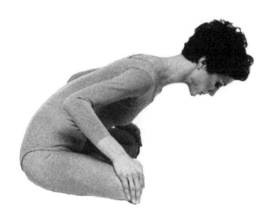

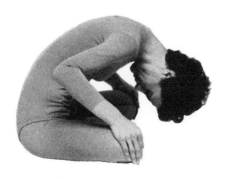

Upper Body (6)

PLACEMENT: Sit with your legs extended as far to the sides as possible, toes pointed, back held erect. Bend the elbows and rest the right hand on top of the left at chest level.

MOVEMENT: Pull the elbows directly back as far as you can, keeping them bent and level. Repeat rapidly ten times. Rest the hands on the knees and roll the head three times to the right, then to the left.

TOTAL REPETITION: Three times.

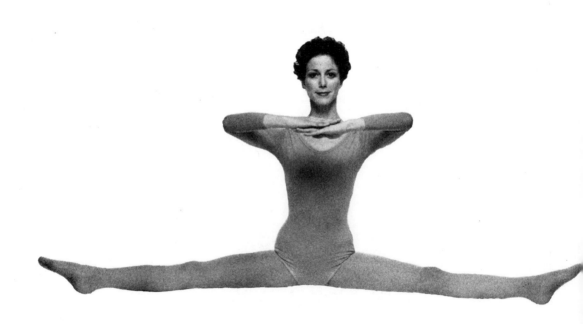

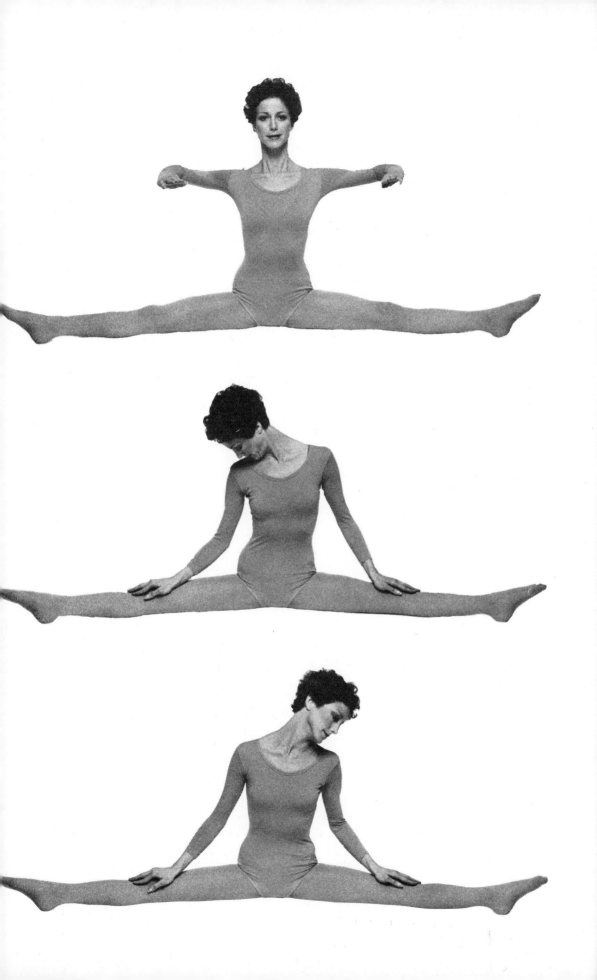

Waist and Abdominals (5)

PLACEMENT: Sit with the legs extended in front, toes pointed, back held erect. Clasp your hands behind your head, elbows open to the sides.

MOVEMENT: Contract your upper body as you lower your head and release your body halfway back until the lower spine touches the floor. The elbows should simultaneously release inward. Hold this position for three counts. Lift the body and open the elbows to the original position. Repeat eight times, then round the back, reach for the ankles, and gently bounce up and down eight times.

TOTAL REPETITION: Two times.

As you release back, remember to tightly contract your buttock muscles.

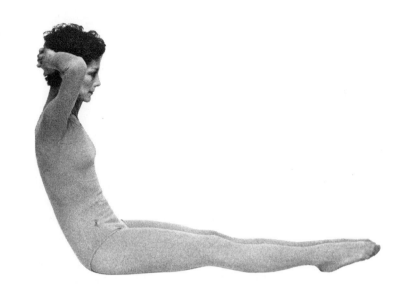

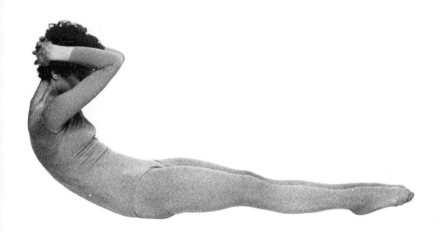

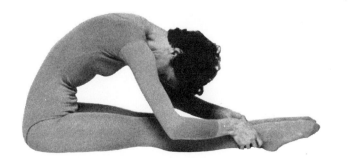

Waist and Abdominals (6)

PLACEMENT: Lie on your back with your knees drawn close to your chest. Rest your hands on your waist.

MOVEMENT: Extend both legs upward until they are straight. Extend them to the sides. Then bring them together before bending them back to the original position. Repeat four times. Pull the knees toward your chest with your hands and hold this position for four counts.

TOTAL REPETITION: Five times.

As you extend your legs, try to keep your abdominal muscles contracted.

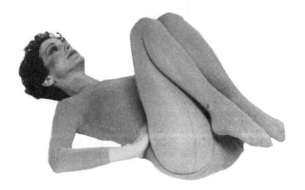

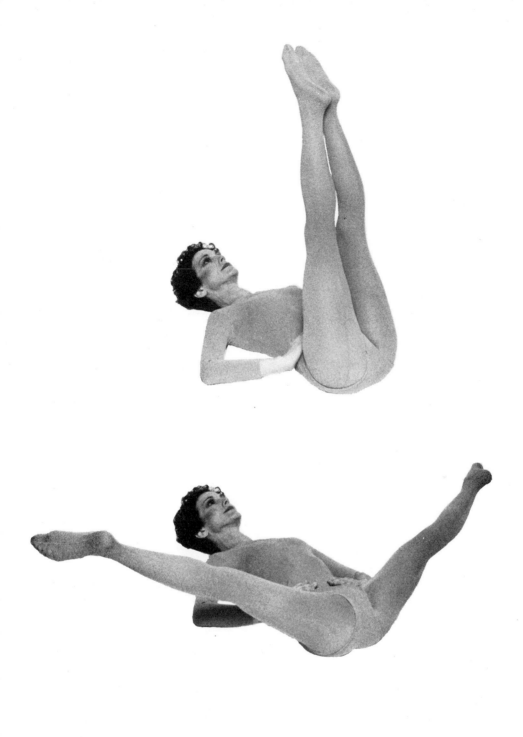

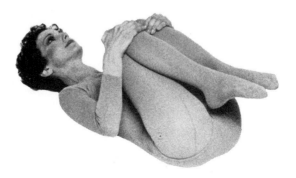

67

Hips and Buttocks (5)

PLACEMENT: Lie on your right side. Lean on your right elbow and keep the torso slightly raised. Use your left hand for additional support. Bend the left leg, drawing the knee close to your chest.

MOVEMENT: In a rapid, sharp motion, straighten and bend the upper leg ten times. Roll over and repeat on the other side.

TOTAL REPETITION: Three times on each side.

By keeping the torso raised, you will also derive a stretch through your waist as well.

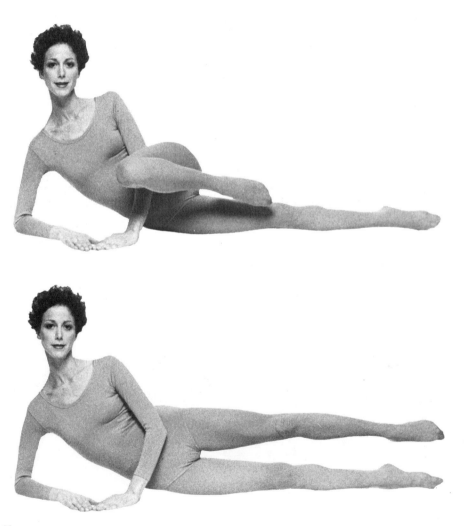

Hips and Buttocks (6)

PLACEMENT: Lie on your back, legs extended in front, heels touching, feet turned out. Rest your hands on your waist.

MOVEMENT: Bend the right leg so that the toes touch the inner part of the left thigh. The outer portion of the right thigh should be close to the floor. Straighten the leg and repeat on the left side.

TOTAL REPETITION: Twenty times.

Keep the abdominals contracted and the buttocks flat on the floor throughout this movement.

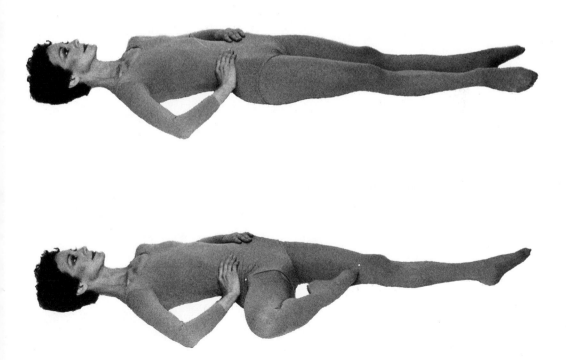

Legs (5)

PLACEMENT: Lie on your back, legs extended in front, toes pointed, hands resting on your waist.

MOVEMENT: Simultaneously lift and cross the right leg to the left side. Lower it to the original position before lifting it to the right side. You are actually forming a "V" with the leg. Repeat four times on each leg.

TOTAL REPETITION: Three times.

As you cross the leg to the side, you will feel the stretch on the outer thigh; as you lift the leg to the side the stretch will be felt on the inner thigh. The wider you form the "V" the more beneficial the exercise will be. Remember to keep your shoulders stationary throughout this movement.

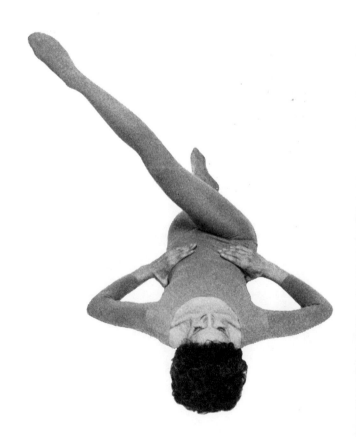

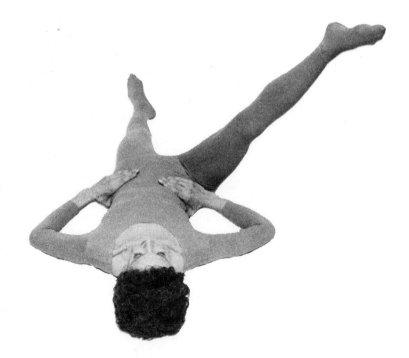

Legs (6)

PLACEMENT: Lie on your back with your left leg bent, sole of the foot on the floor. Extend your right leg upward, toes pointed. Clasp your hands behind the right knee.

MOVEMENT: Pull your leg rhythmically toward your body in a springlike motion. Repeat six times with the foot pointed, then flexed. Repeat on the left leg.

TOTAL REPETITION: Three times on each leg.

This movement not only stretches and tones the hamstring muscle but strengthens the muscles in the lower spine as well.

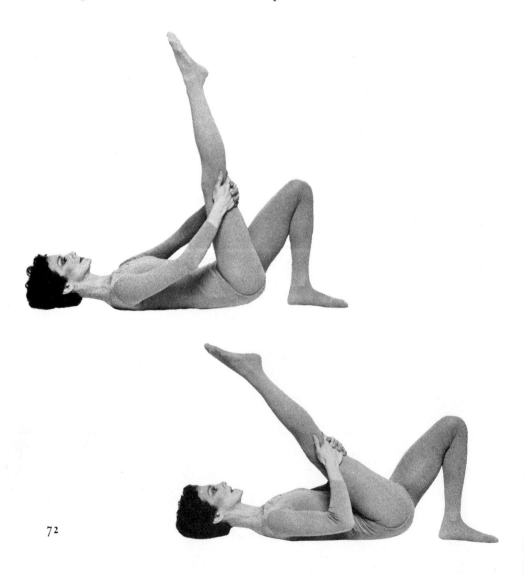

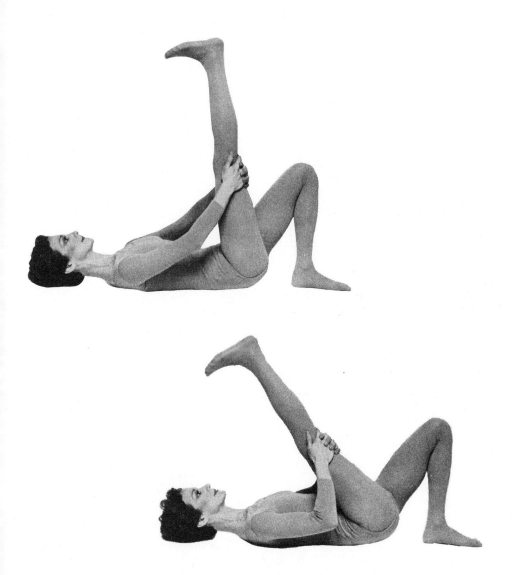

FOURTH WEEK

Upper Body (7)

PLACEMENT: Sit with your legs extended in front, toes pointed, back held erect. Clasp your hands behind your body.

MOVEMENT: Drop the head and round the back as you lift your arms as high as possible. Bounce gently up and down four times, keeping the arms lifted. Lower the arms and straighten your back to the original position.

TOTAL REPETITION: Five times.

Try to prevent your knees from popping up as you lower your body.

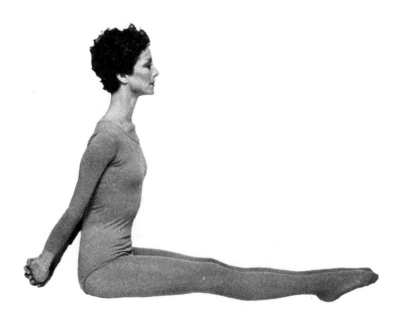

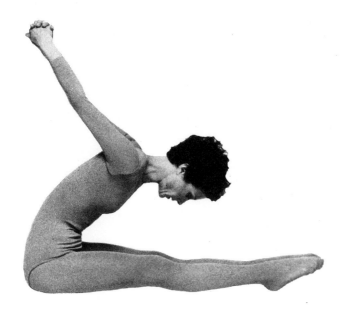

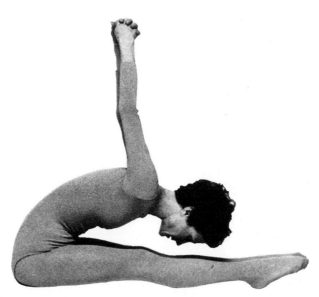

Upper Body (8)

PLACEMENT: Sit with your legs extended to the sides, hands resting on your knees.

MOVEMENT: Round your back and lower your head as close to the floor as possible. At the same time, reach for your ankles. In this position, bounce up and down four times. Uncurl the body slowly until the back is straight.

TOTAL REPETITION: Five times.

Try to keep your head and shoulders relaxed and your abdominals contracted as you bounce.

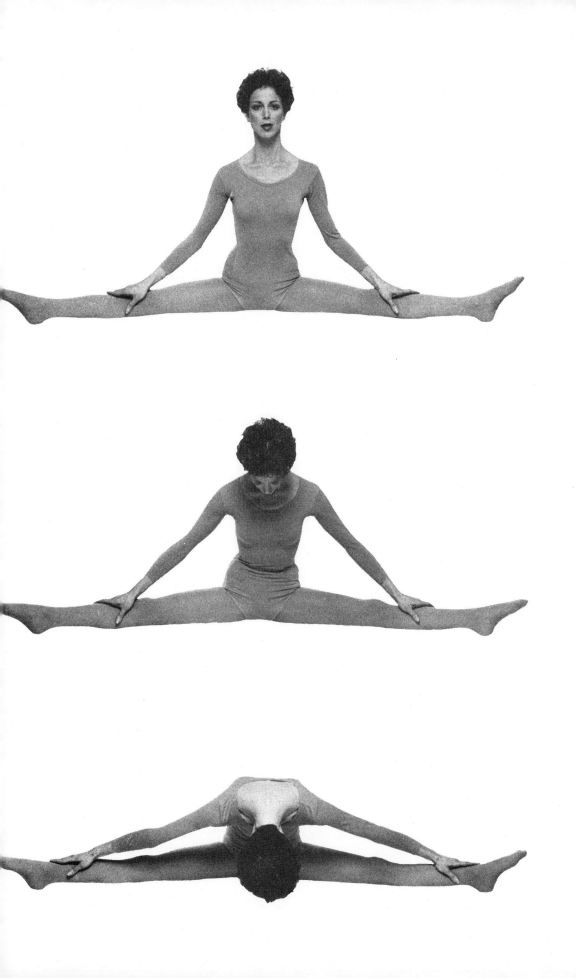

Waist and Abdominals (7)

PLACEMENT: Sit with the knees bent, soles of the feet on the floor. Extend your arms in front at chest level.

MOVEMENT: Contract your abdominal muscles and slowly release your body back until the middle spine touches the floor. Hold this position for three counts, then resume beginning position. Repeat six times. Extend your legs in front, point your toes, and reach for your ankles. Bounce up and down six times.

TOTAL REPETITION: Three times.

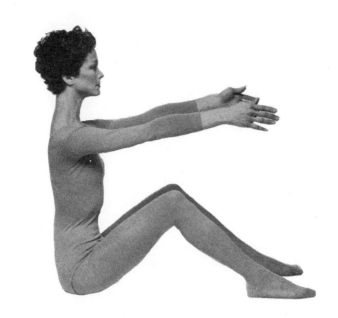

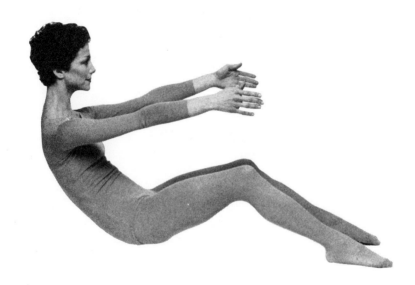

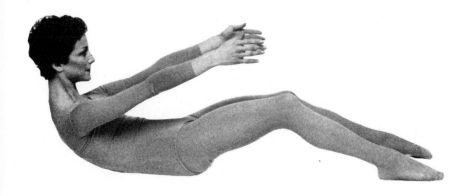

Waist and Abdominals (8)

PLACEMENT: Sit with the right leg extended in front, the foot pointed and turned out. The left leg is bent, the foot resting against the right thigh. Raise the arms overhead and hold the back erect. The shoulders should be directly in line with the hips.

MOVEMENT: Release your torso and reach for your foot with your hands. Bounce gently up and down four times before resuming original position. Repeat five times, then repeat on the left leg.

TOTAL REPETITION: Two times on each leg.

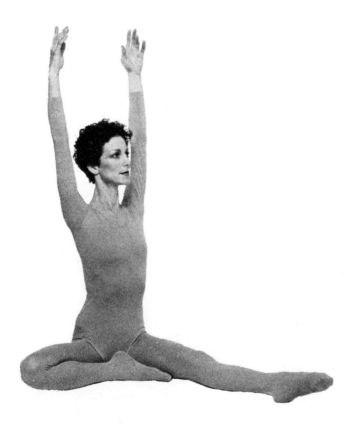

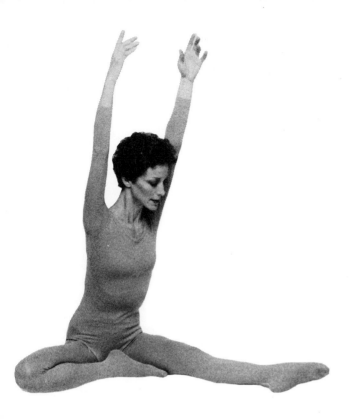

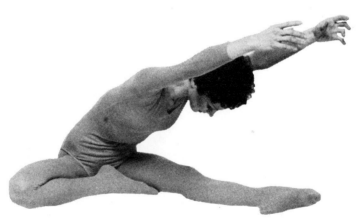

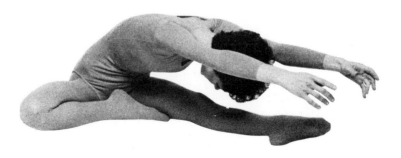

Hips and Buttocks (7)

PLACEMENT: Lie on stomach, arms bent, chin resting on right hand. Legs are together, toes pointed.

MOVEMENT: Grip the buttocks tightly and slowly raise the right leg without turning the body. Lower the leg and repeat on the left side.

TOTAL REPETITION: Twenty-four times.

If your derrière needs toning, this is one of the best movements; try to work up to an eventual fifty leg lifts. Most important, remember to contract the buttocks as you lift the leg and try to keep the hip bone flat on the floor.

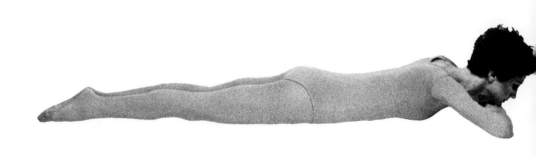

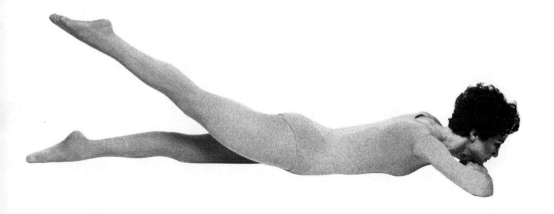

Hips and Buttocks (8)

PLACEMENT: Lie on your right side. Use your right elbow to support your torso, which should be slightly raised. The left hand rests on the floor for additional support.

MOVEMENT: Lift and lower the left leg eight times in a slow, controlled movement, keeping the foot pointed. Roll over and repeat on the other side.

TOTAL REPETITION: Three times on each side.

Try not to lean back on the buttocks as you lift and lower your leg. Instead, lean slightly forward.

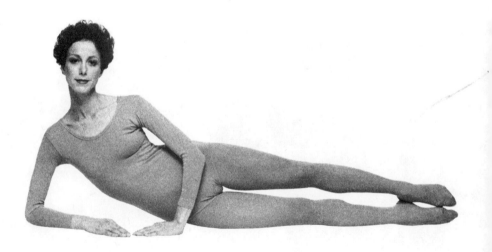

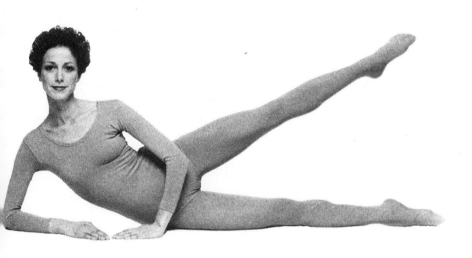

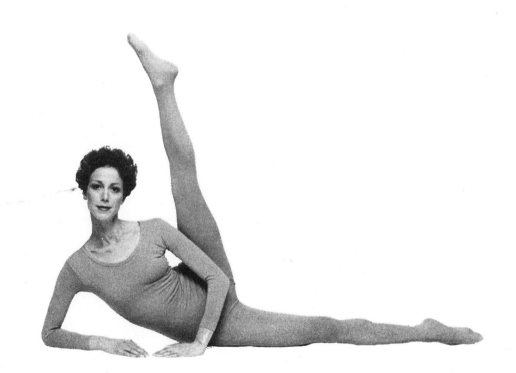

Legs (7)

PLACEMENT: Lie on your back, legs extended in front, toes pointed. Rest your hands on your waist.

MOVEMENT: Form a large, circular movement with your right leg. This is done by crossing the leg to the left, lifting it high and center, extending it out to the side and finally swinging it back to the original position. Repeat five times on the right leg, then on the left.

TOTAL REPETITION: Three times on each leg.

By keeping the foot of the leg that is not moving *turned out*, you will prevent the buttock from lifting off the floor and will thus derive a greater stretch for your waistline as well.

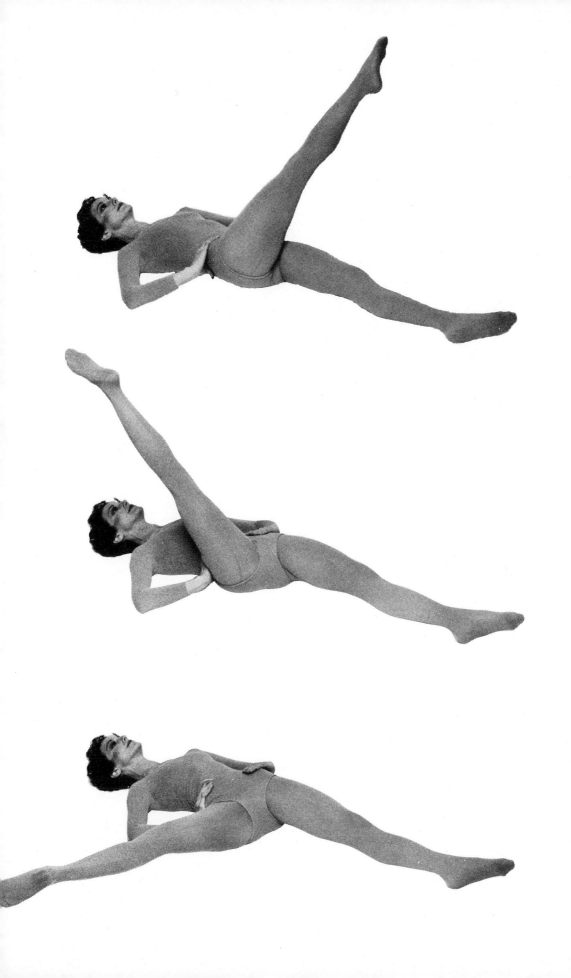

Legs (8)

PLACEMENT: Sit with the soles of your feet together, hands clasped around the toes.

MOVEMENT: Keeping the back erect, bounce the knees up and down twelve times. Lower the head as close to the feet as possible and bounce up and down six times. Uncurl slowly, beginning with the lower spine, until the back is straight.

TOTAL REPETITION: Four times.

This exercise will strengthen your inner thigh muscles so that you are able to sit with your legs extended to the sides with greater ease and agility.

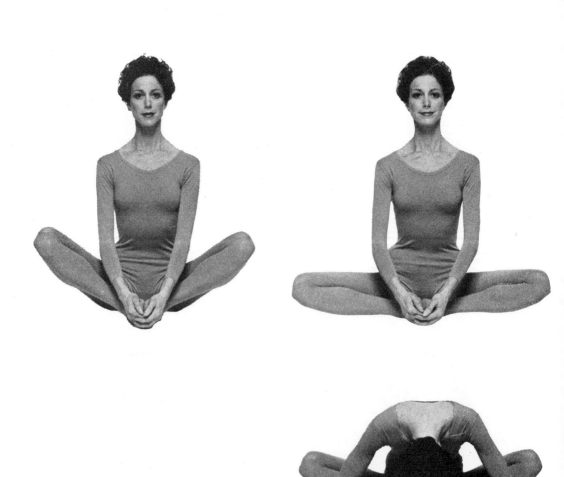

FIFTH WEEK

Upper Body (9)

PLACEMENT: Lie on your stomach, legs together, toes pointed. Rest your forehead on the floor and clasp your hands behind your body.

MOVEMENT: Lift the arms as high as possible without straining or forcing the movement. Take three slow counts to lift and three to lower.

TOTAL REPETITION: Ten times.

If you contract your buttock muscles as you lift the arms, you will derive additional benefits from this exercise.

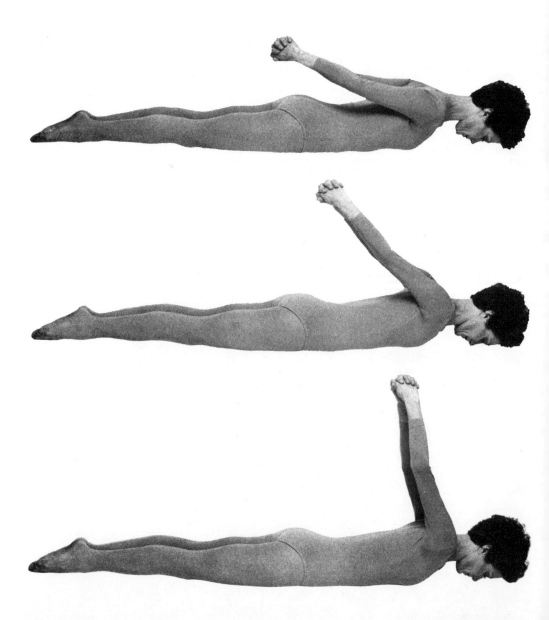

Upper Body (10)

PLACEMENT: Lie on your back with your knees drawn close to your chest. Your head should rest in your hands, which are clasped together, elbows touching the floor.

MOVEMENT: Lift your head, neck, and shoulders off the floor, bringing your elbows together. Take three counts to lift and three to release.

TOTAL REPETITION: Twelve times.

Inhale as you lift the body, exhale as you release.

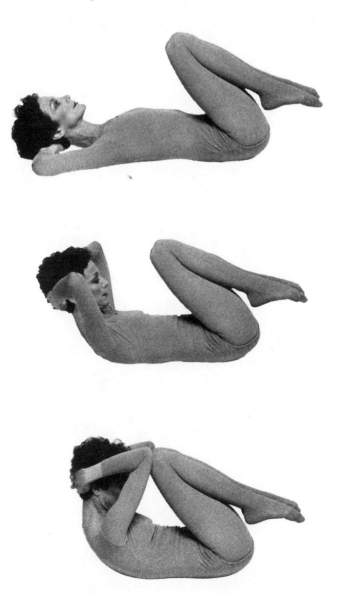

Waist and Abdominals (9)

PLACEMENT: Sit with legs extended to the sides, toes pointed, arms extended upward.

MOVEMENT: Alternating arms, stretch and reach higher and higher (as if you were climbing a rope) eight times. Round the back, rest your palms on the floor, and bounce up and down eight times. Uncurl slowly to the original position.

TOTAL REPETITION: Three times.

Remember to keep your abdominals contracted as you reach overhead. If executed properly, you should feel this stretch from your arms to your waist.

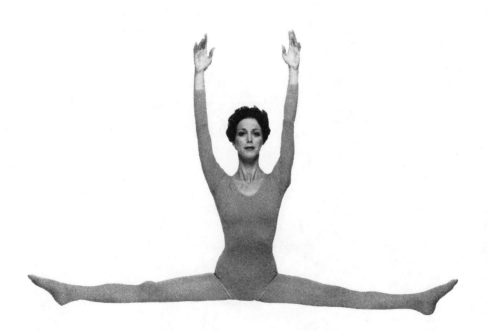

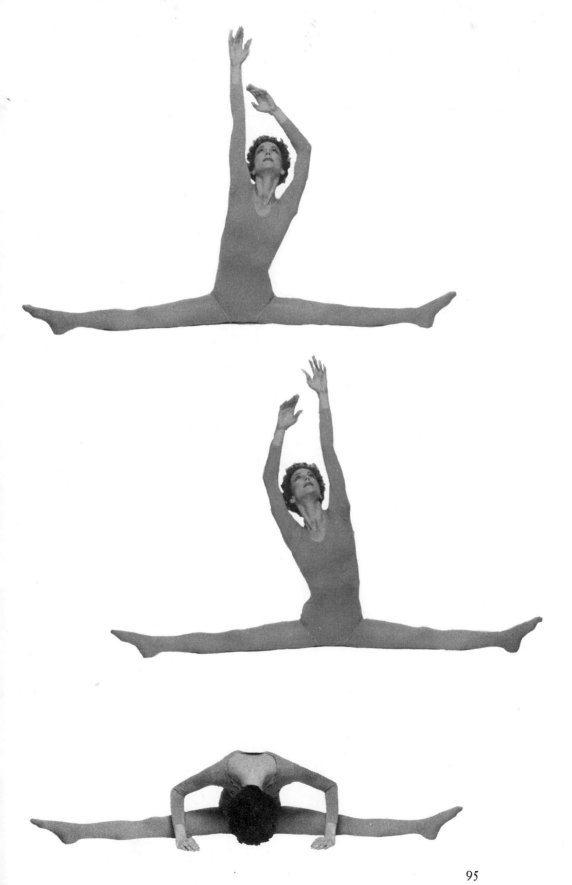

Waist and Abdominals (10)

PLACEMENT: Lie on the floor, left leg extended in front, right knee drawn close to your chest. Clasp your hands around the knee and lift your head, neck, and shoulders off the floor.

MOVEMENT: Keeping the upper body raised, lift and lower the left leg four times. Release the head to the floor and draw both knees to your chest, hold for three counts. Repeat with the right leg.

TOTAL REPETITION: Two times on each leg.

If you find this movement too difficult, it can also be done without lifting the upper body off the floor. Practice it in this manner until you are more comfortable with the exercise.

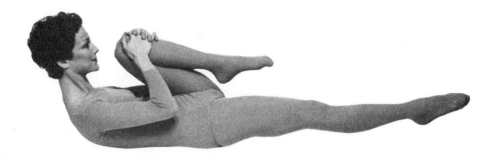

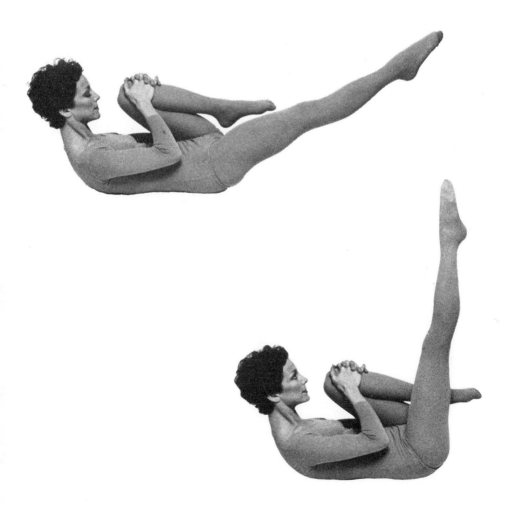

Hips and Buttocks (9)

PLACEMENT: Lie on your back with the knees bent, feet parallel and about ten inches apart. Rest your arms at your sides, palms facing down.

MOVEMENT: Contract the buttock muscles tightly and slowly raise the body as high off the floor as you can. In this lifted position, bounce gently up and down four times. Uncurl back to the floor, beginning with the upper back. The buttocks should touch the floor last. Take four counts for each part of this movement. Repeat six times, then draw the knees to your chest and hold for six counts.

TOTAL REPETITION: Two times.

As you release from the lifted position, remember to contract your abdominals and grip the buttocks. The uncurling process must be very controlled so that your spine is totally flat before the buttocks touch the floor.

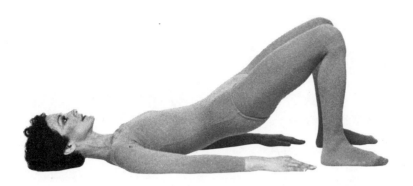

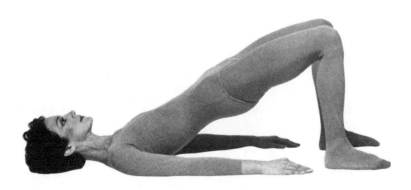

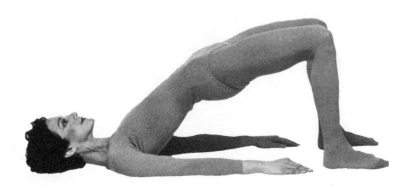

Hips and Buttocks (10)

PLACEMENT: Lie on your stomach, elbows bent, chin resting on top of right hand. The legs are together, toes pointed.

MOVEMENT: Lift the right leg as high as possible without turning the body or bending the knee. In this raised position, bounce the leg up and down three times. Lower it to the floor and repeat with the left leg.

TOTAL REPETITION: Ten times.

As you lift the leg, tighten the buttock muscles and keep them contracted until you begin to lower the leg to the floor.

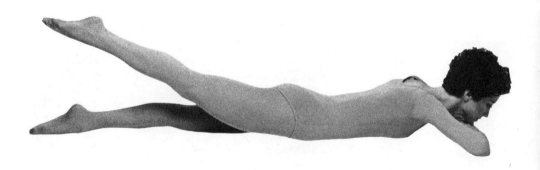

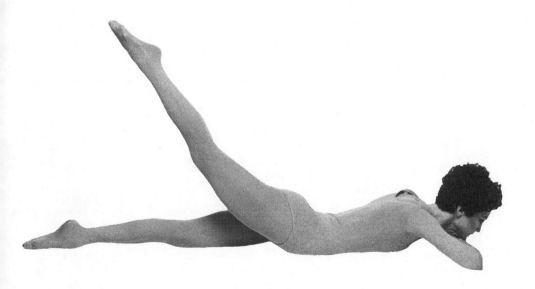

Legs (9)

PLACEMENT: Lie on your back, both legs extended upward, toes pointed. Rest your hands on the inner part of the leg, close to the calf.

MOVEMENT: Gently force the legs apart with your hands and bounce them in this extended position four times before resuming the original position. Repeat five times, then bend the knees, drawing them to the chest, and hold for eight counts.

TOTAL REPETITION: Four times.

This is one of the most effective movements for firming the inner thighs. Remember to keep your abdominals contracted as you bounce the legs up and down in order to prevent your back from arching. You can also bounce the legs with the feet in a flexed position—alternate if you wish.

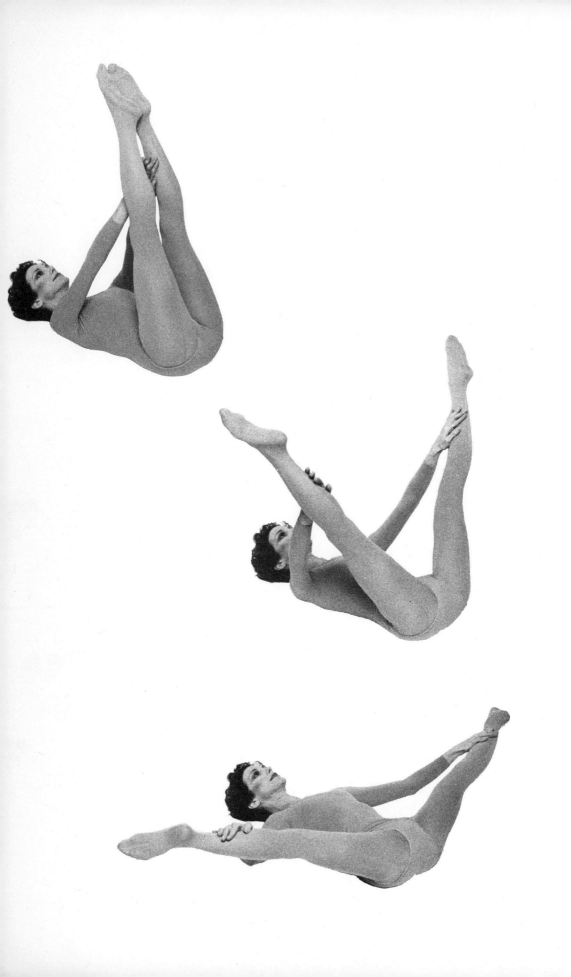

Legs (10)

PLACEMENT: Sit with the left leg bent, foot close to the body. Clasp your hands around the right ankle. Point the toes so they are just touching the floor.

MOVEMENT: Keeping the back as erect as possible, extend the right leg until it is straight. Repeat six times, then repeat with the left leg.

TOTAL REPETITION: Three times on each leg.

If you find it is too difficult to extend the leg with your hands on the ankle, try clasping them higher up on your leg—near the calf. Although it is impossible to keep the back totally straight as you extend the leg, try not to lean back unnecessarily.

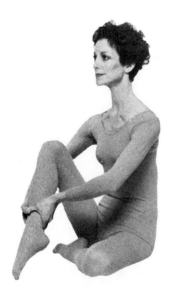
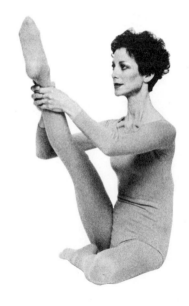

SIXTH WEEK

Upper Body (11)

PLACEMENT: Sit with your legs extended to the sides, toes pointed, back erect. Clasp your hands behind your body.

MOVEMENT: Release your torso over the right leg as the arms simultaneously lift. Pull the arms down as you lift the body and repeat to the left side.

TOTAL REPETITION: Sixteen times.

For this movement to be most effective, try to keep your buttocks as stationary as possible as you lower your torso. Keep your abdominals pulled in and your legs straight throughout.

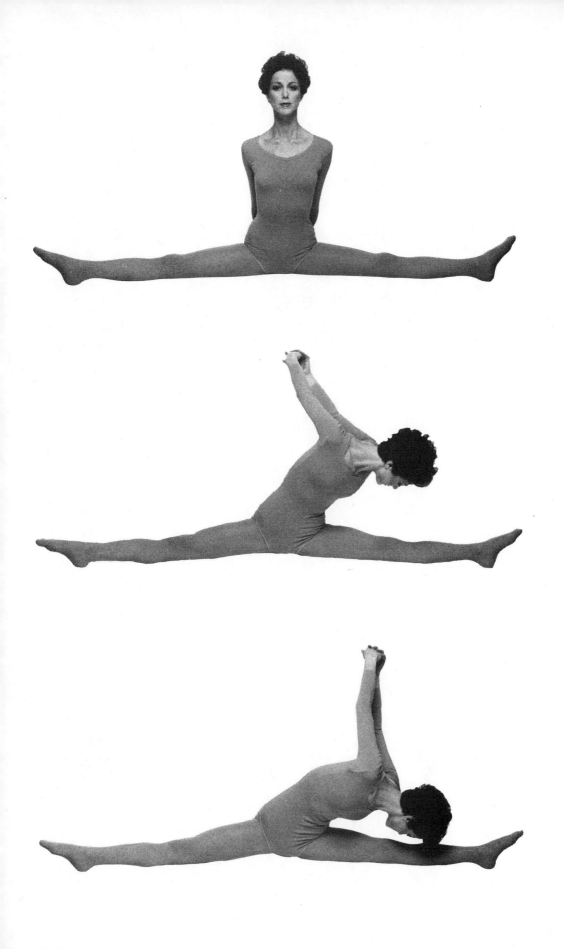

Upper Body (12)

PLACEMENT: Lie on your stomach, elbows bent, chin resting on top of the right hand. Legs are together, toes pointed.

MOVEMENT: Slowly open the arms to the side as you gently arch your upper body and grip your buttock muscles. Release and rest for three slow counts before repeating.

TOTAL REPETITION: Eight times.

This movement, if done properly, without forcing, should be felt in the chest, not in the lower back. There is no need to overly arch the back in order to derive benefits from this exercise.

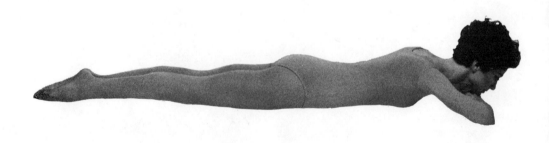

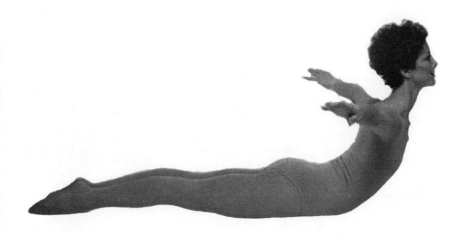

Waist and Abdominals (11)

PLACEMENT: Sit with legs extended to the sides, toes pointed, arms relaxed.

MOVEMENT: Twist the torso from the waist and try to clasp both hands as close to the right ankle as you can. Gently bounce up and down five times, keeping the buttocks flat and the abdominals contracted. Repeat to the left side.

TOTAL REPETITION: Four times on each side.

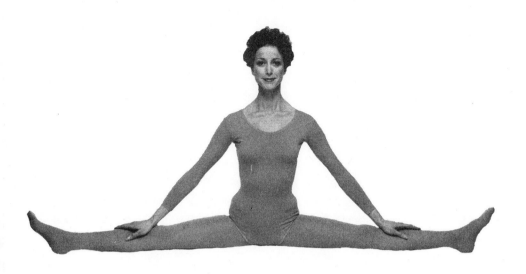

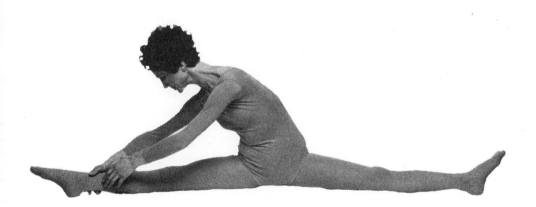

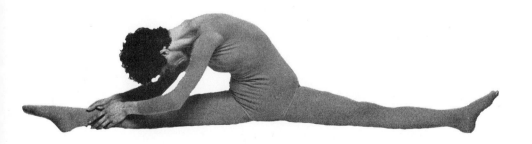

Waist and Abdominals (12)

PLACEMENT: Lie on your back with your legs extended in front, toes pointed, arms resting at your sides.

MOVEMENT: Raise your head, neck, shoulders, and arms off the floor until your upper and middle spine are no longer resting on the floor. At the same time, bend your knees until the soles of your feet are flat on the floor. Hold this contraction for three slow counts, keeping the abdominals pulled in throughout. Release slowly to the original position.

TOTAL REPETITION: Ten times.

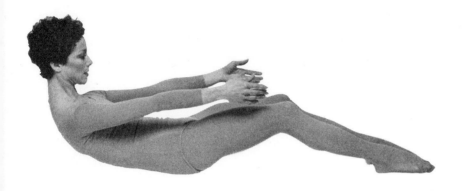

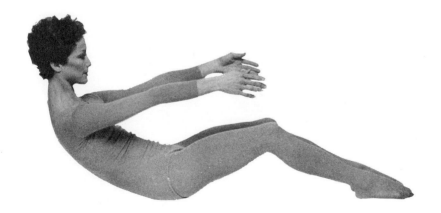

Hips and Buttocks (11)

PLACEMENT: Lie face down, elbows bent, chin resting on right hand. Keep your legs together and straight, toes pointed.

MOVEMENT: Lift the right leg off the floor, swing it to the right side, return it center, and lower it to the original position.

TOTAL REPETITION: Twenty-four times.

As you swing the leg to the side, be sure to keep it high and straight. Also remember to contract the buttock muscles throughout this movement.

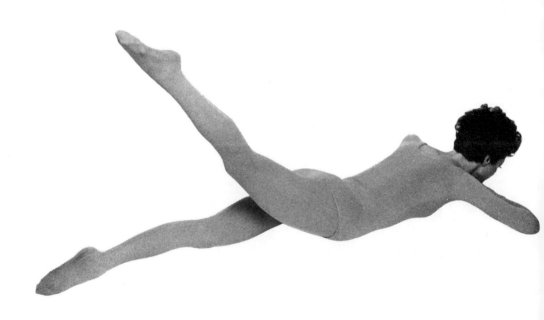

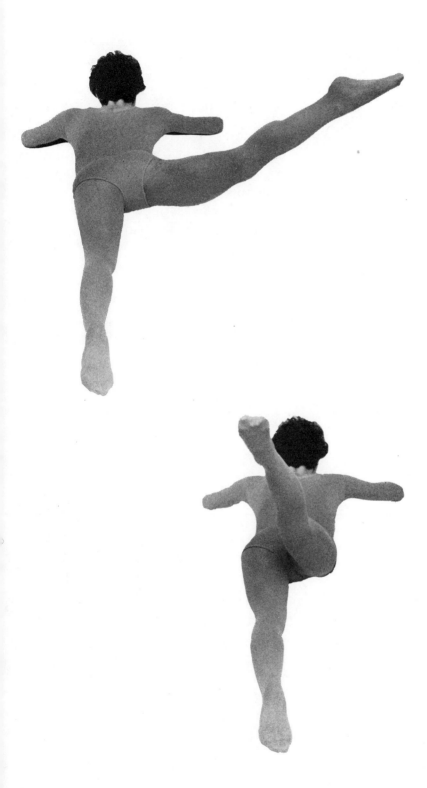

Hips and Buttocks (12)

PLACEMENT: Lie on your back, knees bent, feet parallel and about ten inches apart. Rest your arms at your sides, palms facing down.

MOVEMENT: Contract your buttock muscles and slowly raise your body as high off the floor as you can. At the same time, lift the arms and lower them to the floor overhead, palms facing up. In this raised position, gently tilt the hips and buttocks from side to side six times. Lower the arms as you slowly uncurl the body, beginning with the upper back, until you have resumed the original position. Remember, the buttocks are last to touch the floor.

TOTAL REPETITION: Four times.

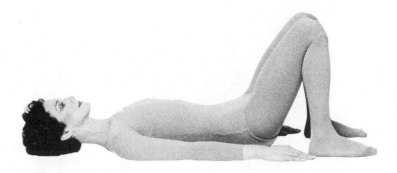

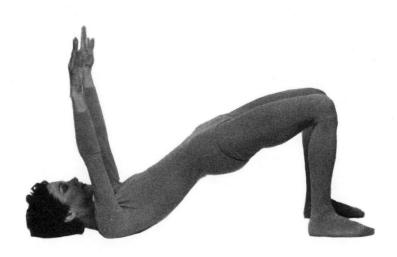

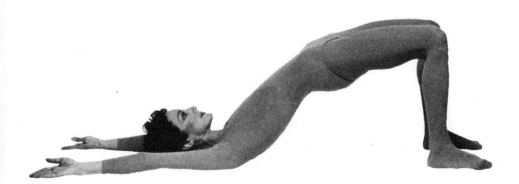

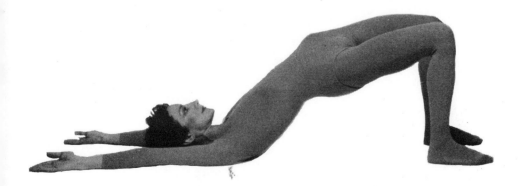

Legs (11)

PLACEMENT: Lie on your right side, using your right elbow to support your torso, which should be slightly raised. Place your left hand on the floor for additional support. Bend the left leg and rest the toes on the right thigh.

MOVEMENT: In a quick, rhythmic motion, straighten and bend the leg twelve times, keeping the toes pointed throughout. Roll over and repeat on the other side.

TOTAL REPETITION: Three times on each side.

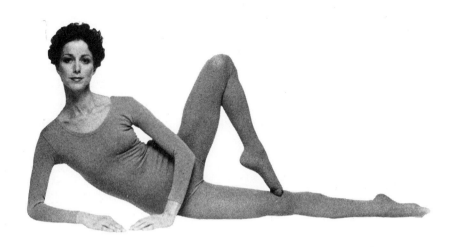

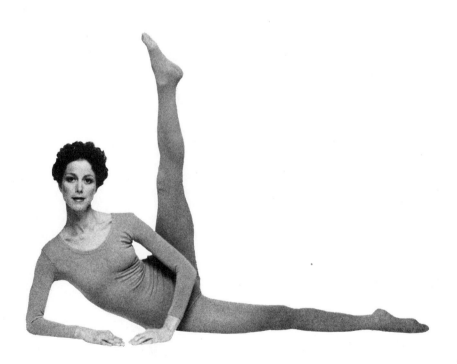

Legs (12)

PLACEMENT: Lie on your back, knees drawn close to your chest, arms at your sides.

MOVEMENT: Straighten your legs upward by supporting your hips and buttocks with your hands. Slowly release the legs overhead, keeping them totally straight, until your toes touch the floor. Relax your arms at your sides and hold this position for about thirty seconds. Slowly uncurl the back, until it is flat and the legs are extended directly overhead. Bend the knees to the original position and relax for ten counts.

TOTAL REPETITION: Two times.

As you develop more and more strength and flexibility in your back, you will be able to sustain the position for longer periods of time. If you are unable to hold the position for thirty seconds, work up to it gradually.

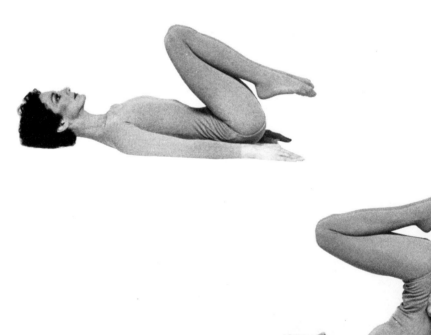

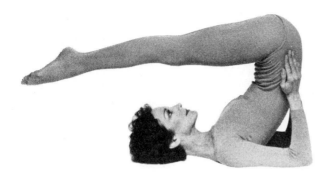

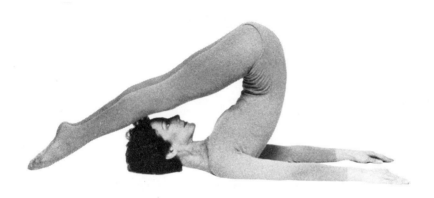

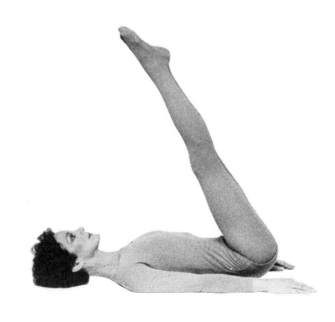

SEVENTH WEEK

Upper Body (13)

PLACEMENT: Sit on floor with the soles of your feet together, chin lifted, arms stretched overhead.

MOVEMENT: Alternating arms, stretch overhead (as though you are climbing a rope) six times. Release the arms, round the back, and clasp your ankles. Bounce up and down six times.

TOTAL REPETITION: Four times.

As you reach overhead, keep your abdominals pulled in and your back as erect as possible. You should feel this stretch in your waist as well as in the upper arms. Try to separate your torso from your hip area as you stretch.

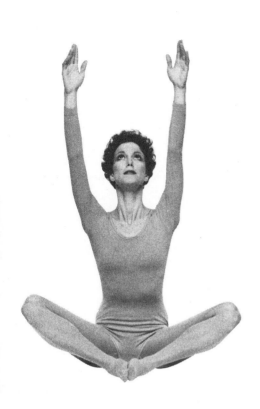
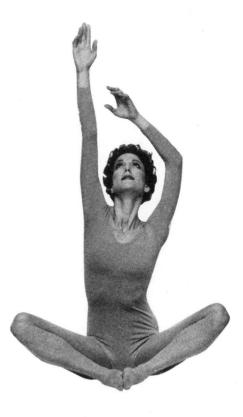
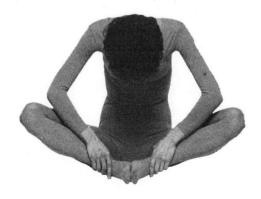
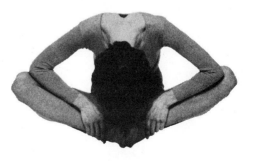

Upper Body (14)

PLACEMENT: Sit with the ankles crossed, hands resting on your knees.

MOVEMENT: Contract the torso, round the shoulders, and drop the head as close to the floor as possible. Flatten the back by lifting the head and pulling the shoulders back. Straighten the body to the original position. Take two slow counts for each part of this movement.

TOTAL REPETITION: Twelve times.

This exercise should be done with an even, steady motion. There should be no pausing at any point in the movement.

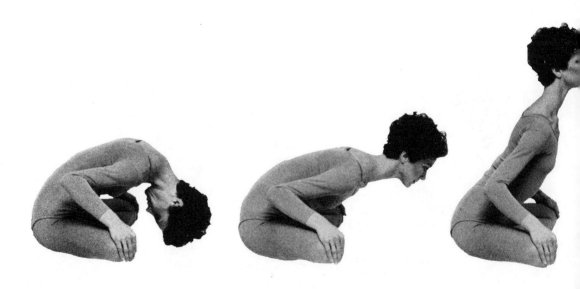

Waist and Abdominals (13)

PLACEMENT: Sit with both legs extended in front. Rest hands on your hips and release the body back until the lower spine is touching the floor. Contract the abdominals and point the toes.

MOVEMENT: Alternating legs, lift and lower them four times. Release the body over the legs and reach for your toes. Hold this position for four counts.

TOTAL REPETITION: Five times.

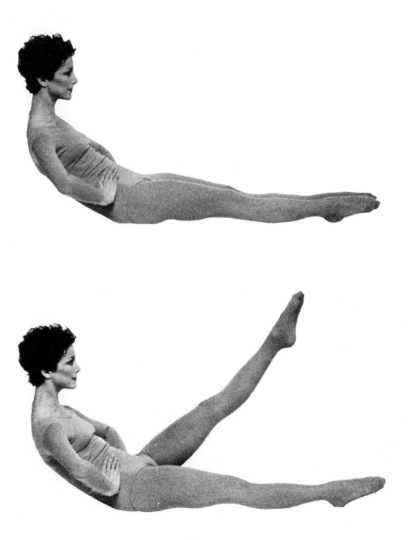

Waist and Abdominals (14)

PLACEMENT: Sit with your legs extended as far to the sides as possible, toes pointed. Rest your hands on your legs.

MOVEMENT: Lean and stretch your torso to the right as your right hand reaches toward the right foot and your left arm arches overhead, palm facing up. Repeat to the left side.

TOTAL REPETITION: Twenty-four times.

This stretch should be done slowly in order to be most effective. The objective is to bring the side of your head as close to the leg as you can. Try to keep the buttocks as flat as possible and the legs straight throughout.

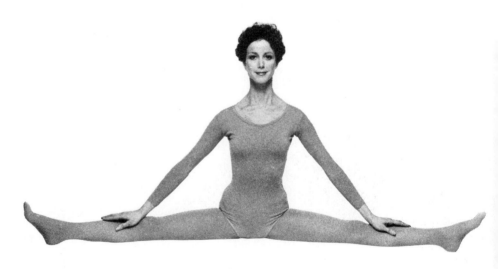

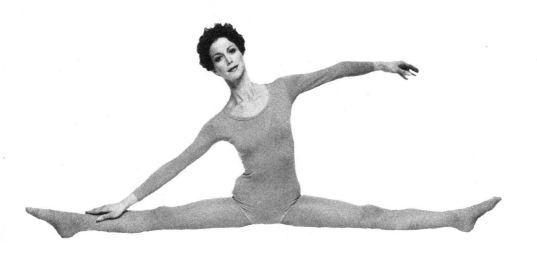

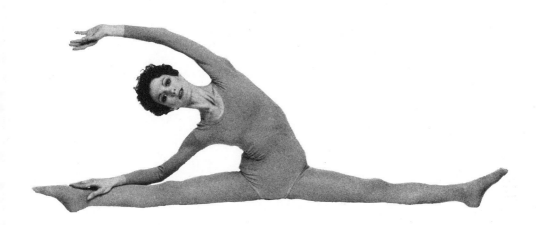

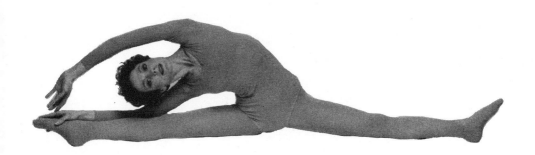

Hips and Buttocks (13)

PLACEMENT: Lie on the floor with the right leg extended upward, toes pointed, left leg extended on the floor. Arms rest on the floor at shoulder level, palms facing down.

MOVEMENT: Keeping the shoulders flat throughout, cross the right leg to the left side and as close to the floor as possible. Bounce it up and down four times. Return the leg to the upward extended position before slowly lowering it to the floor. Repeat on the left leg.

TOTAL REPETITION: Eight times.

This is an excellent exercise for the waistline as well—be sure to keep the shoulders stationary.

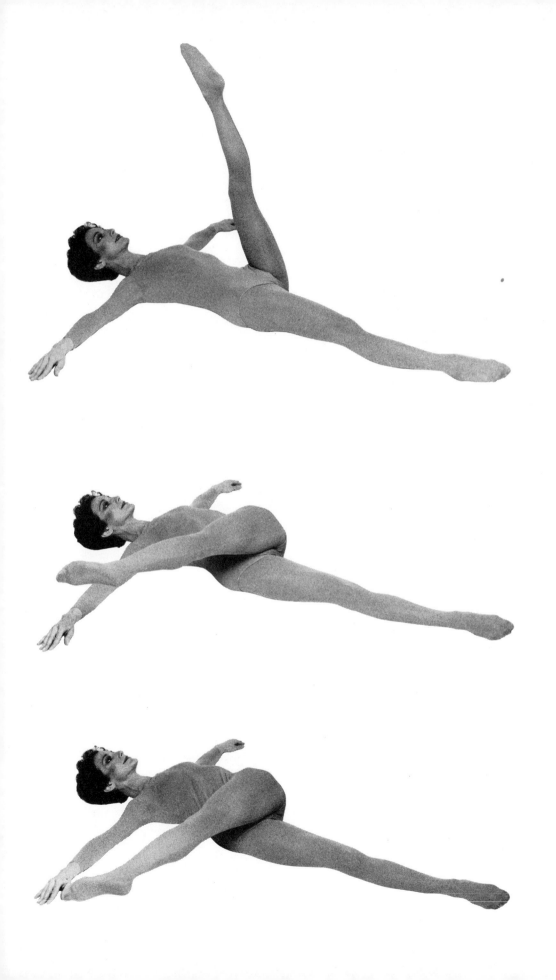

Hips and Buttocks (14)

PLACEMENT: Lie on your back, legs extended in front, toes pointed, feet turned out. Rest your hands on your waist.

MOVEMENT: Bend the right leg so that the toes touch the inner portion of the left thigh. Extend the leg to the side until it is straight and slightly raised off the floor. Swing it back into place and repeat on the left leg.

TOTAL REPETITION: Twenty-four times.

Be certain to keep the foot of the straight leg turned out in order to prevent your buttock from lifting off the floor.

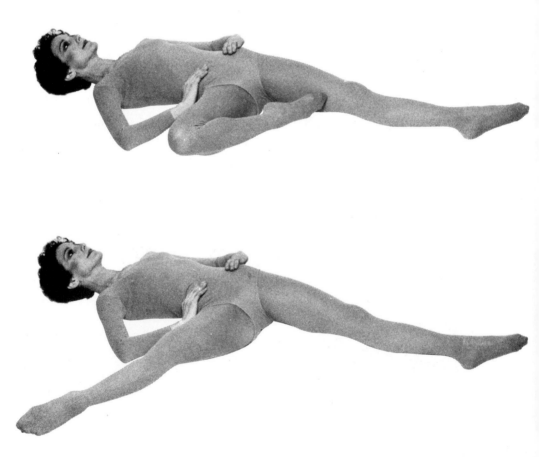

Legs (13)

PLACEMENT: Kneel on the floor with the knees about twelve inches apart.

MOVEMENT: Reach back and grasp your ankles with both hands. Rock back and forth four times keeping the abdominals and buttocks tightly contracted. Release the ankles and push yourself forward to the original position.

TOTAL REPETITION: Five times.

The majority of the stress should be placed on the abdominals and the front of the thighs. Avoid arching the back as much as possible.

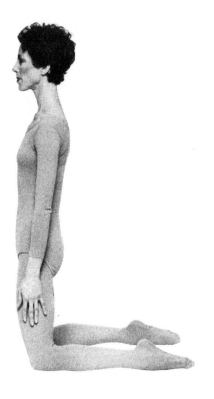
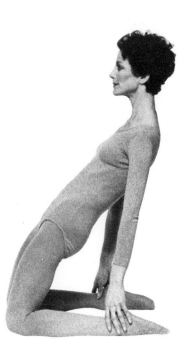

Legs (14)

PLACEMENT: Sit on the floor and grasp your heels with your hands. Rest your toes on the floor and your elbows on your legs. The knees should be open to the sides.

MOVEMENT: Extend your legs to the sides until they are straight, then bend them to the original position. Repeat six times at a moderate tempo. Cross your ankles, rest your hands on your knees, and lower your head as close to the floor as you can. Hold this position for six counts.

TOTAL REPETITION: Four times.

In order to best maintain your balance, make certain to keep your abdominals contracted as you extend your legs to the sides.

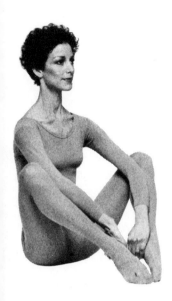

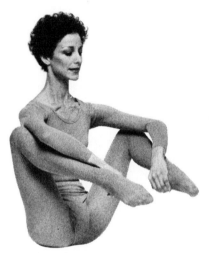

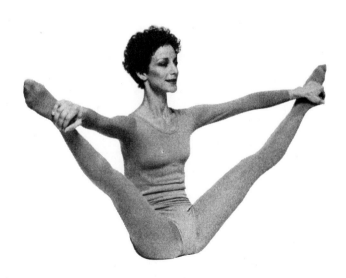

EIGHTH WEEK

Upper Body (15)

PLACEMENT: Sit with the right leg extended to the side. Bend the left leg and place the foot close to the body. The shoulders should be directly in line with the hips.

MOVEMENT: Lean and stretch your torso to the right. Reach for your right foot with the right hand as the left arm arches overhead, palm facing up. Keep the left buttock flat on the floor. Bounce gently up and down five times before resuming the original position. Repeat four times, then change positions and repeat to the left side.

TOTAL REPETITION: Three times to each side.

As you stretch to the side, try to bring the side of your head as close to the leg as you can. This is a wonderful stretch for the waistline as well as the upper arms.

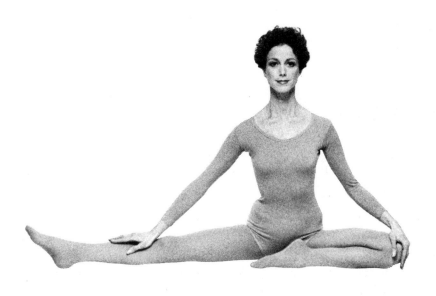

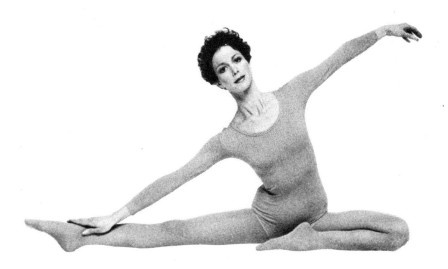

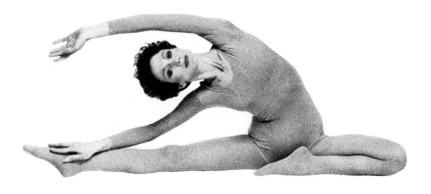

Upper Body (16)

PLACEMENT: Lie on your back with the right leg extended in front. Bend the left leg and rest the foot on the floor. Extend the arms overhead on the floor, palms facing up.

MOVEMENT: Swing the arms forward and down to the floor at your sides, palms facing down, as the head, neck, and shoulders lift off the floor. At the same time, the right leg lifts toward the body. Hold for three counts, then release to the original position. Repeat five times, then change and repeat on the left leg.

TOTAL REPETITION: Two times on each side.

The objective is to bring the lifted leg as close to the body as possible without bending the knee.

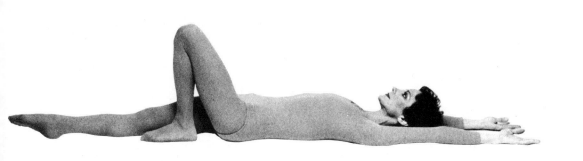

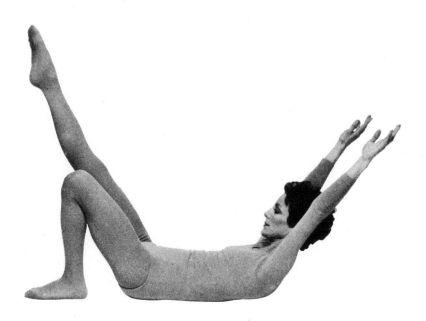

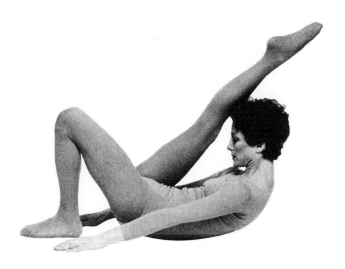

Waist and Abdominals (15)

PLACEMENT: Sit with your knees bent, soles of the feet resting on the floor and about twelve inches apart. Rest your hands on top of your knees.

MOVEMENT: Contract your abdominals, release your body halfway back, keeping the soles of your feet on the floor. Your arms simultaneously lift overhead. Hold this position for three counts before returning to original position. Repeat four times. Cross your ankles, place your hands on the floor, and bounce gently up and down four times, bringing your head as close to the floor as possible.

TOTAL REPETITION: Four times.

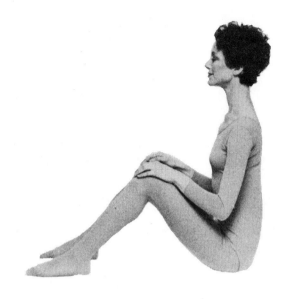

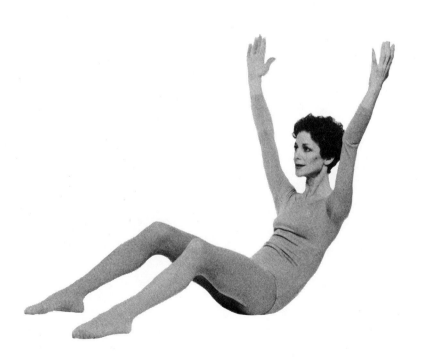

Waist and Abdominals (16)

PLACEMENT: Sit with your knees bent, toes pointed and just touching the floor. Lean back slightly, raise your arms upward, palms facing in.

MOVEMENT: Extend the legs until they are straight, then resume original position. Repeat fairly rapidly six times. Stretch the legs on the floor, drop your head, round your back, and reach for your ankles. Hold this position for six counts.

TOTAL REPETITION: Four times.

If you are unable to sustain your balance while extending your legs, support yourself by placing your fingertips on the floor at your sides. The key to maintaining your balance is to contract your abdominals as you straighten your legs.

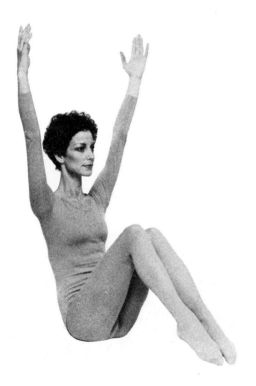
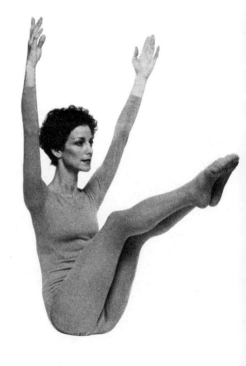

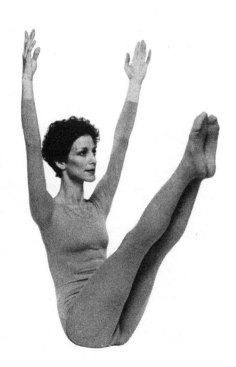

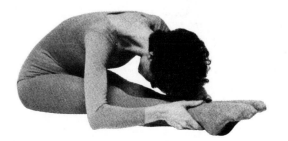

Hips and Buttocks (15)

PLACEMENT: Lie on your right side. Lean on your right elbow, keeping the torso slightly raised. Rest your left hand on the floor in front of your body for additional support. Bend the left knee and draw it close to your chest.

MOVEMENT: Thrust the left leg back until it is straight, gripping the buttocks as you do so. Resume original position and repeat eight times. Roll over and repeat on the other side.

TOTAL REPETITION: Three times on each side.

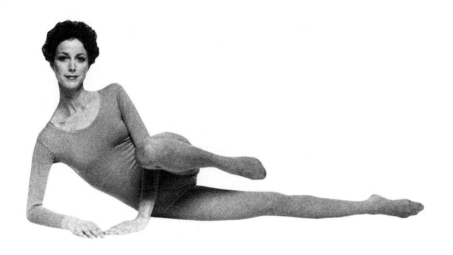

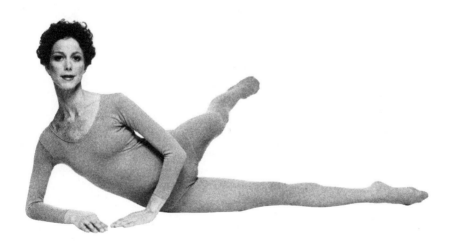

Hips and Buttocks (16)

PLACEMENT: Lie on the floor, arms extended at shoulder level, palms facing down. Extend the right leg upward, toes pointed. The left leg is extended on the floor, the foot turned out.

MOVEMENT: Keeping the left foot turned out, swing the right leg as far to the left, then as far to the right as you can, without bending the knee. Repeat four times, then return the leg center before lowering it slowly to the floor. Repeat with the left leg.

TOTAL REPETITION: Three times on each leg.

Remember to keep the foot that is not raised turned out and the shoulders stationary. The swinging leg should be raised as high as possible.

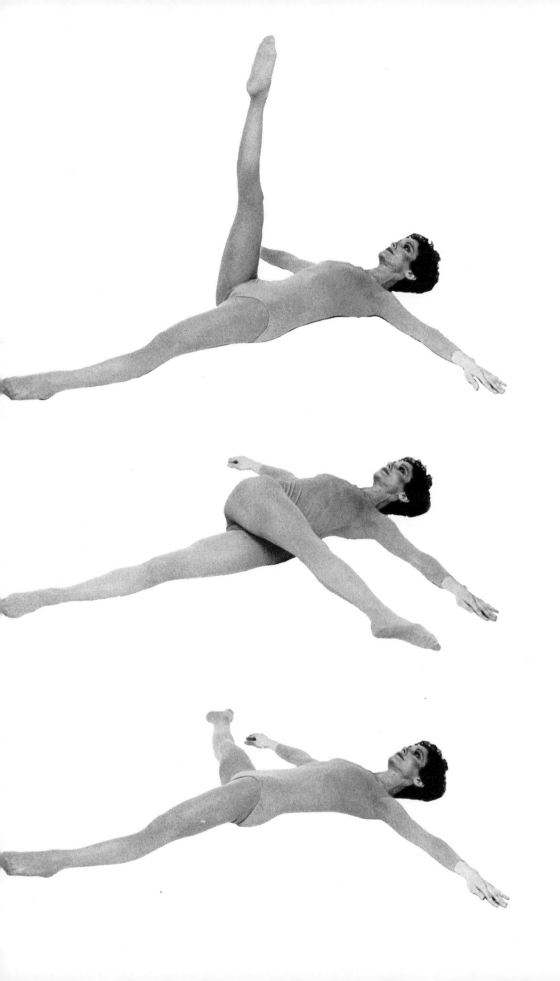

Legs (15)

PLACEMENT: Kneel on the floor, arms extended in front at chest level, knees about twelve inches apart.

MOVEMENT: Contract the buttock and abdominal muscles and slowly release the body back as far as you can without overly arching the back. Resume the original position by slowly lifting forward until your back is erect.

TOTAL REPETITION: Eight times.

If you are unable to repeat this movement eight times, work up to it gradually since it requires strong abdominal and thigh muscles. Do not tilt your head backward. By doing so you will place too much stress on your neck muscles.

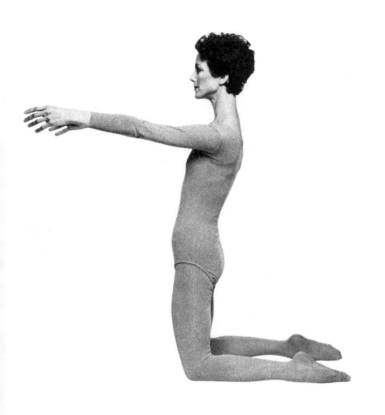

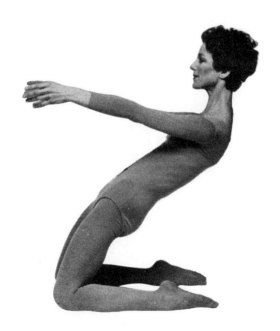

Legs (16)

PLACEMENT: Lie on your back, right leg extended upward, left leg on the floor. Clasp your hands on the right leg near the calf.

MOVEMENT: Release your grip on the right leg and lower it until the foot is practically touching the floor. Simultaneously raise your left leg and pull it toward your body. The hands should rhythmically change from one leg to the other as each is pulled toward the body. Alternate ten times. Draw the knees to your chest and hold this position for ten counts. Perform the same scissor-like movement with the legs, this time with your head, neck, and shoulders lifted off the floor.

TOTAL REPETITION: Two times in each position.

Try to keep the legs as straight as possible and the toes pointed throughout this exercise.

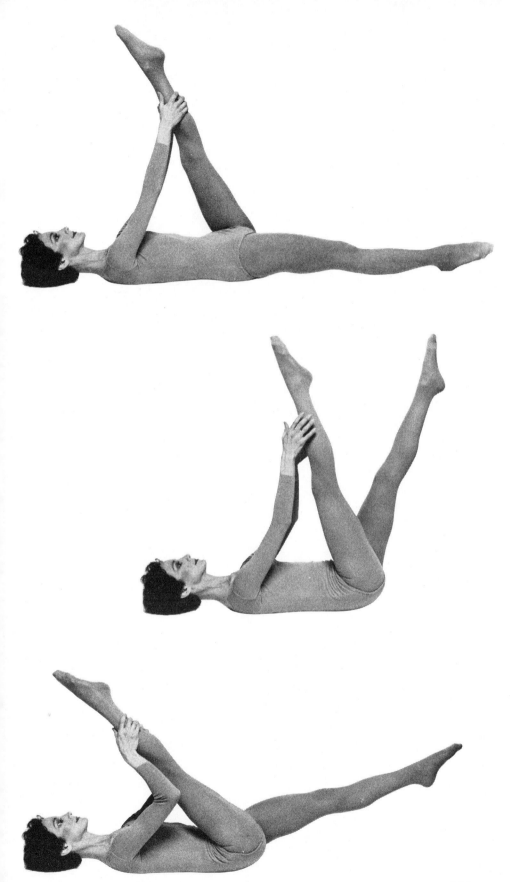

Pregnancy and Postnatal Recovery

A woman who is in good shape before pregnancy usually reaps the benefits throughout the nine months, as well as during her post-natal recovery. Her energy and stamina are bound to be higher and she will have a "reservoir" of endurance which is so necessary at that time. The pregnant woman owes it to herself (and indirectly to the baby) to maintain the best tone and shape she possibly can. Although pregnancy is not the time to begin a new and rigorous sport or exercise regimen, a woman need not remain inactive. Naturally, activities will have to be somewhat curtailed or modified, since you're apt to fatigue more readily. Nevertheless, if you're in good health and have your doctor's approval to exercise, you can remain relatively active. Most dancers continue to take classes through their final weeks of pregnancy and generally experience easy deliveries. This is undoubtedly a result of their superb muscle tone and overall fitness.

In the more advanced stages of pregnancy, many women experience lower back pains—often for the first time in their lives. This is generally due to their additional weight combined with weak muscles or poor postural habits. During pregnancy, the curve of the lower spine naturally increases in order to balance the protruding abdomen. This can often cause back discomforts of varying degrees. Since pregnancy does place stress on the lower spine, a woman (in order to counteract this) should concentrate on maintaining the best possible postural habits. She should exercise regularly in order to maintain strength in the supporting muscles of the back. If you're pregnant and suffering from back discomfort, make certain to devote a minimum of ten minutes a day to the Back Strengthening exercises in this book. Once the pains begin to lessen, you'll be convinced how important these exercises truly are.

It has been my experience that most women are able to continue practicing the majority of the movements in this program throughout their pregnancy. Many of the exercises actually resemble those taught in the

Lamaze natural childbirth classes. Movements performed while sitting on the floor, either with the legs extended to the sides (page 79) or with the soles of the feet together (page 81), are particularly effective as preparation for labor. Only those exercises that require you to lie on your stomach should be eliminated in the final months. If, however, you are uncomfortable doing some of the more advanced movements, choose only those that you can perform with ease and confidence.

Providing you haven't gained an excessive amount of weight during the nine months, you should have little trouble regaining your normal weight and figure. Naturally, no matter how well-toned you were prior to your pregnancy, your abdominals are bound to be somewhat flaccid afterward. That's nature's way of allowing the muscles to stretch in order to accommodate a full-term baby. Don't despair or become discouraged; most women regain their tone within a mere few weeks once they begin to exercise regularly. When your physician gives you the go-ahead to begin doing some gentle, nonstrenuous exercises (many encourage this after about ten days or so), you may start with any of the Postpregnancy exercises, Back Strengtheners or Relaxercises. Spend only a few minutes at first, choosing those exercises you feel most comfortable with. Avoid overextending the sessions (begin with about five minutes and work up to more) or straining your body in order to achieve extreme positions. Be certain to curb your enthusiasm. Spend about two weeks (more if you wish) on only these exercises. Then, when you feel ready for a more concentrated regimen, begin with the less demanding movements in the program. You might even decide to follow the entire eight-week program from beginning to end. If you begin to tire before the fifteen minutes are completed, reduce the time to best suit your needs. Always remember to take the signals from your body, since pushing yourself will only retard your progress.

Post-pregnancy Shape-Up (1)

PLACEMENT: Sit with the ankles crossed. Extend the arms in front at chest level, palms facing in.

MOVEMENT: At a moderate tempo, open the arms as far to the sides as possible, without forcing. Repeat eight times. Shake out the arms and repeat same movement with the palms facing out.

TOTAL REPETITION: Two times.

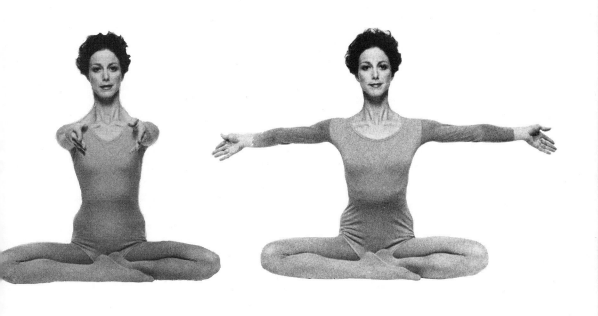

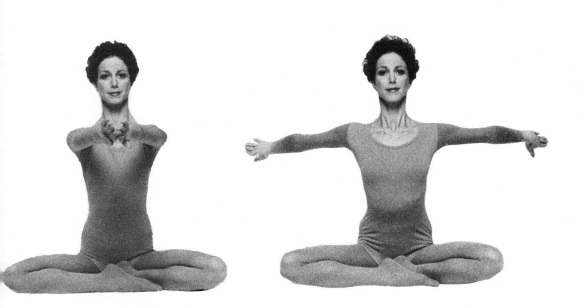

Post-pregnancy Shape-Up (2)

PLACEMENT: Lie on your back, left leg extended on the floor, right leg drawn close to your chest with your hands.

MOVEMENT: Slowly lift your head, neck, and shoulders off the floor as you pull your knee closer to your chest. Hold for three counts, then release the head to the floor. Repeat five times, then repeat with the left leg.

TOTAL REPETITION: Two times on each leg.

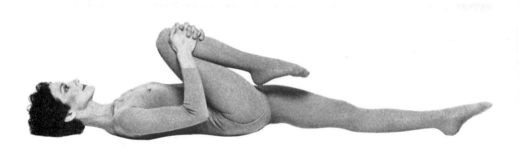

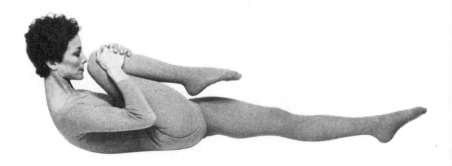

Post-pregnancy Shape-Up (3)

PLACEMENT: Lie on your back. Rest the left foot on the floor, extend the right leg in front. Hands rest on your hips.

MOVEMENT: Lift and lower the right leg ten times. Repeat on the left.

TOTAL REPETITION: Three times on each leg.

As you lift and lower the leg, contract your abdominals and press your spine against the floor.

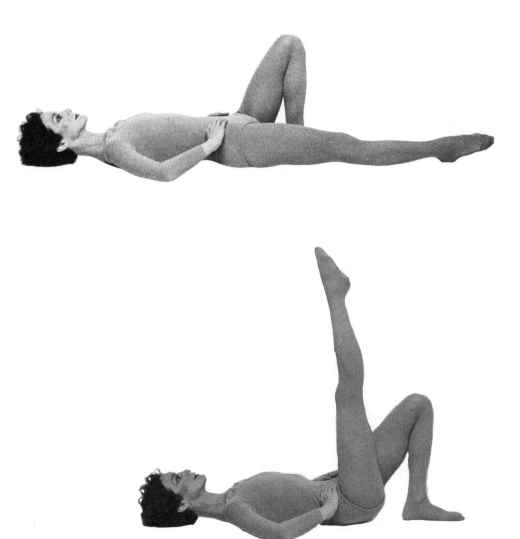

Post-pregnancy Shape-Up (4)

PLACEMENT: Lie on the floor with the arms extended at shoulder level, palms facing down. Draw the knees to your chest.

MOVEMENT: Keeping the knees together and the shoulders stationary, roll the knees from side to side. Try to lower them as close to the floor as you can.

TOTAL REPETITION: Twelve times.

This exercise will help to shape and firm your waistline. Remember to flatten the back against the floor each time when knees return to center position.

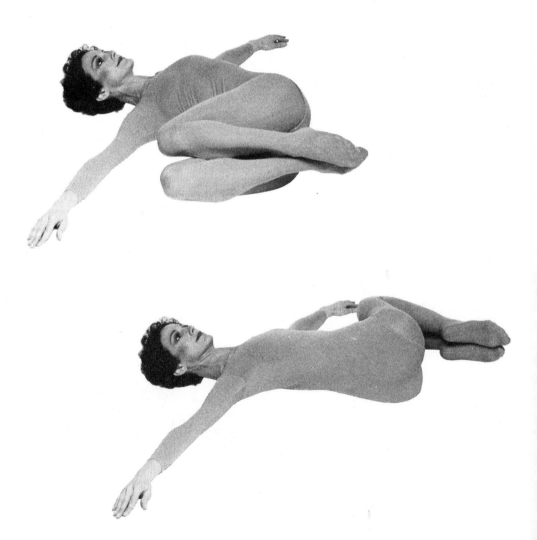

Post-pregnancy Shape-Up (5)

PLACEMENT: Sit on the floor with your legs extended in front, arms raised overhead.

MOVEMENT: Round the back, drop the head, and reach for your toes. Bounce gently up and down four times, keeping your abdominals contracted. Resume original position and stretch overhead, alternating arms, four times.

TOTAL REPETITION: Five times.

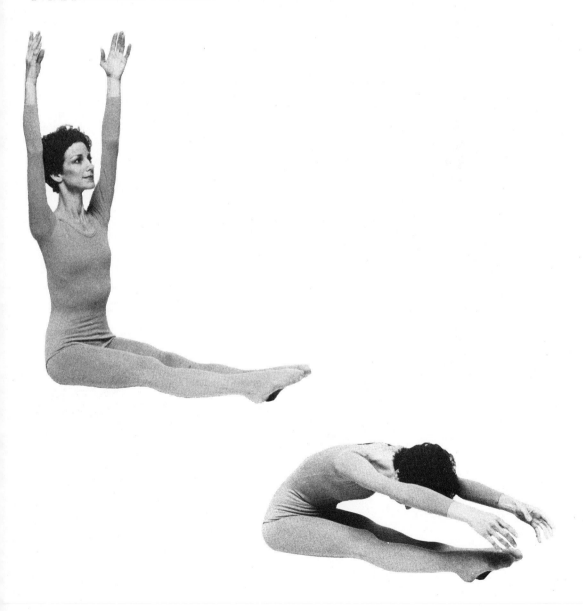

Post-pregnancy Shape-Up (6)

PLACEMENT: Sit with legs extended in front, hands resting on waist.

MOVEMENT: Contract your abdominals and release your body halfway back until your lower spine touches the floor. Hold this position for three counts, then lift to original position. Repeat six times. Round the back, reach for your toes, and gently bounce up and down six times.

TOTAL REPETITION: Two times.

As you release back, remember to tightly grip your buttock muscles as well as your abdominals.

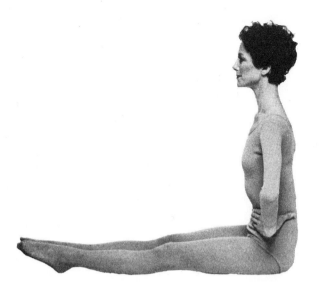

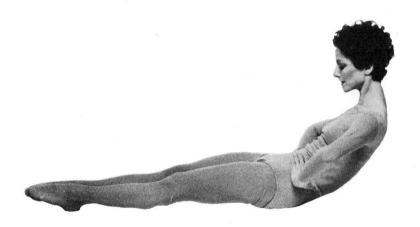

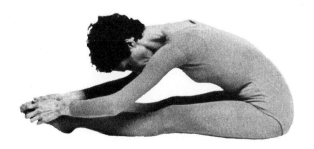

Backaches and Pains

Although many of the exercises in this program develop tone, strength, and flexibility of the spine, it is so important and crucial an area that I have devoted an entire section to back-strengthening movements of an orthopedic nature. The health and condition of your back greatly affects your overall fitness. When the back is pained, you cannot function at your best. Back pains result from numerous factors; sometimes it is simply a case of inflexibility where muscles are not fully stretched to give the full range of movement needed. Many back discomforts are caused by stress and tension. The most common causes, however, are poor postural habits and inadequate exercise. By abusing the back (holding it out of line) or neglecting it (robbing it of exercise), the muscles that support the spine become weak and lose their elasticity.

When your back is strong and held erect, you will invariably sit, stand, and move with greater ease. Almost naturally, the rest of your body (head, shoulders, abdomen, etc.) falls into line. Figure flaws are also so much more obvious when one's posture is incorrect. No matter what a woman's age or bone structure might be, if her body alignment is correct, she can look more graceful and attractive. To hold the body properly is simply a matter of training your mind to command your body and your body to obey the commands. Although there are numerous reasons for poor posture, the most common is plain laziness. Granted it's going to take a conscious effort to correct improper postural habits if you've been negligent for years, but once they're eliminated, the posture problem is solved.

Common early morning back pain can generally be lessened significantly (or totally eliminated) with what I call the "Cat Stretch." If you've ever observed a cat when it first awakens from a nap, you might have noticed how it slowly stretches in a somewhat exaggerated manner. This same sort of stretching can work for you to prevent morning stiffness from lingering all day. Before you get out of bed, treat yourself to a minute or two of *total* stretching from head to foot. Get all the kinks and stiffness out of your joints. Actually, it's really quite unreasonable to expect your body to spring into action with the buzz of your alarm clock. Try to make it a point to begin the day with a total stretch.

Regular practice of the movements in this program can help diminish back discomforts of many kinds. One of my clients, a dentist, complained of general pain and discomfort through his shoulders, neck, and upper back. This was undoubtedly the result of the tense and awkward positions he assumed during the course of his working hours. As soon as he adopted the habit of stretching and limbering up between patients, the strain he experienced disappeared. The back-strengthening exercises that I have included in this chapter are those that will stretch tight, stiff back muscles, as well as strengthen other muscles (such as the abdominals) so that they too can share the work load that would otherwise be assumed only by the back. If you suffer from back pains and aches, these exercises will prove extremely beneficial—providing you do them regularly. This means spending approximately ten minutes a day on the simple but effective movements in this section.

Back Strengthener (1)

PLACEMENT: Lie on your back with your knees bent, soles of the feet on the floor. Rest your arms at your sides.

MOVEMENT: Contract your abdominals and press your spine against the floor. Hold the contraction for eight slow counts, then release.

TOTAL REPETITION: Eight times.

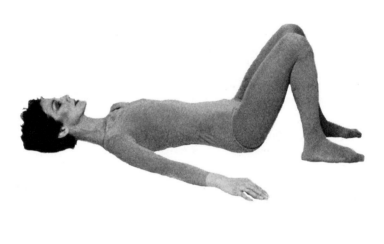

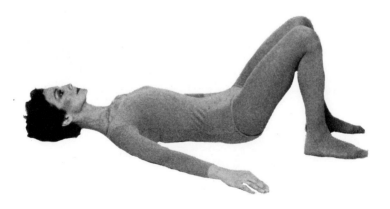

Back Strengthener (2)

PLACEMENT: Lie on your back, head resting in clasped hands, elbows touching the floor. Bend the knees and rest the soles of the feet on the floor, about ten inches apart.

MOVEMENT: Lift your head, neck, and shoulders off the floor as you bring your elbows together. Rock forward and back gently three times before releasing to the original position. Relax for three counts.

TOTAL REPETITION: Six times.

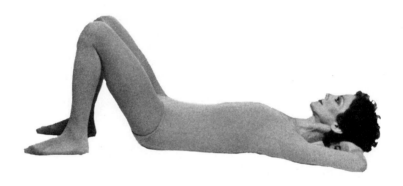

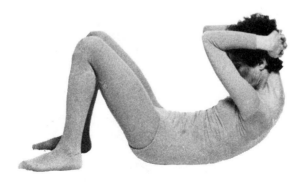

Back Strengthener (3)

PLACEMENT: Sit with ankles crossed, hands resting on the knees, back erect.

MOVEMENT: Round the back and lower the head as close to the floor as possible. Gently bounce up and down four times, keeping the abdominals contracted. Uncurl slowly to the original position.

TOTAL REPETITION: Six times.

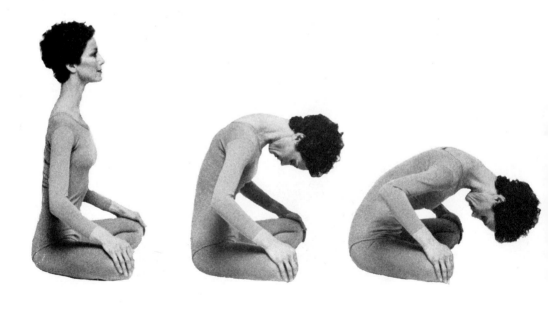

Back Strengthener (4)

PLACEMENT: Lie on your back, knees bent, feet parallel and about ten inches apart.

MOVEMENT: Clasp your hands around the right knee and pull it toward your chest in a back-and-forth movement ten times. Repeat on the left leg.

TOTAL REPETITION: Three times on each leg.

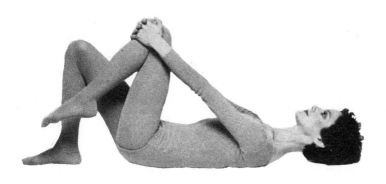

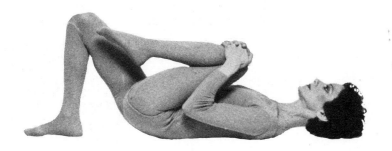

Back Strengthener (5)

PLACEMENT: Lie on your back with your legs extended upward. Clasp your hands behind the knees.

MOVEMENT: In a steady, gentle motion, pull the legs toward your body five times. Bend the knees and draw them toward your chest, hold for five counts.

TOTAL REPETITION: Five times.

Try to keep the toes pointed and the legs as straight as possible as you pull them toward you.

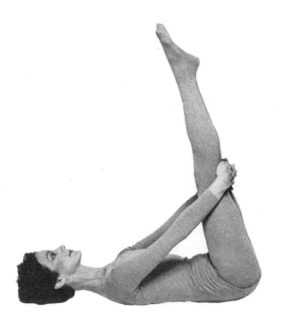

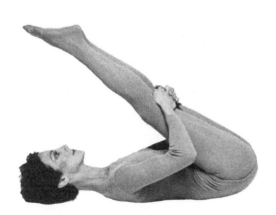

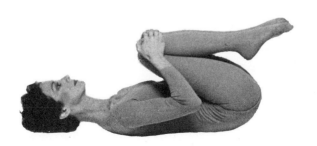

Back Strengthener (6)

PLACEMENT: Lie on your back, legs extended in front, arms stretched overhead and resting on the floor.

MOVEMENT: Contract your abdominals, pressing the spine against the floor. At the same time, bend your knees slightly. Hold the contraction for five counts, then release.

TOTAL REPETITION: Ten times.

A more advanced version of this exercise is to flatten your back against the floor without bending the knees at all.

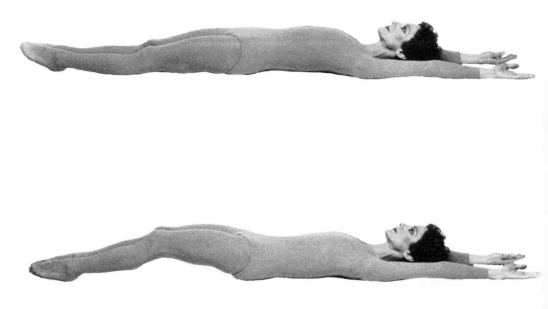

Stress and Exercise

We are all subject to tension of one kind or another, perhaps not daily, but enough so that it takes its toll on both the mind and body. The next time you feel tense and upset, check to see exactly how you've reacted, since mental and physical strain can truly rob you of vital energy that might otherwise be utilized far more productively. In what way does stress manifest itself for you? Have you tightened your neck and shoulders? Has your stomach gone into a spasm? Which muscles have actually assumed the brunt of the tension? Try to stop in your tracks and pinpoint exactly which areas have been affected. By breaking muscle behavior patterns, you can actually diminish the amount of strain and stress you experience. For instance, if, whenever you feel upset, your upper back and shoulders become rigid, try some simple shoulder rotations (page 176) or the overhead stretching motion with your arms raised high (page 27). Should you feel a headache developing, spend a few minutes on the Deep Breathing exercise which is absolutely ideal for calming and easing the nerves. Remember, you need not lie down to do the breathing exercise; it can be done while sitting, standing, or even walking.

It's sometimes difficult to make yourself move when you're tired or tense. It's even a chore to *think* about exercising. You'll discover again and again, however, that it's well worth the initial effort. Taking time out for a regular stretch regimen will actually help you develop a greater capacity to deal with upsetting situations. You will not only feel more relaxed as you do the slow, controlled movements (especially if you use some soothing music), but you'll attain a sense of relaxation that will last well after your practice session is completed. Many of my clients have found that after a frenetic day, spending a few minutes on just the Relaxercises (simple positions designed for the express purpose of easing the mind and relaxing the body) can revitalize them for the remainder of the evening.

When I'm weary, but haven't the time to actually nap, I close my bedroom door, turn off the lights, and take several minutes out for the following exercise: Lie on the floor with your arms at your sides and your legs extended in front. Try to withdraw your mind from problems and thoughts of your surroundings by concentrating only on your muscles. Begin by tightening your muscles until you feel totally rigid and stiff. Then, let go and relax each and every muscle. Begin with the tip of your toes. Relax your feet, legs, and thighs. Next relax your back, shoulders, arms, hands, even your fingertips. Let the muscles of your neck and face relax as well. Imagine that your body is melting into the floor—I like to think of myself as a weightless, fluffy powderpuff. Remain in this serene state for a few minutes, completely at ease and calm. When you're finally ready to sit up, rise slowly. Stretch and yawn and enjoy the sensation of feeling tranquil and relaxed, I frequently recommend this muscle-releasing exercise to my clients who find they're too "wound up" to fall asleep at night. It really does work quite beautifully. Learning to relax and "let go" is actually discovering one of the most important secrets to attaining a healthy, productive life.

Relaxercises (1)

Sit on the floor with the ankles crossed. Stretch your arms on the floor in front of your body, elbows bent, palms facing down. Relax the head. Hold this position for about one minute. Inhale deeply and uncurl the body slowly. Repeat as many times as you wish.

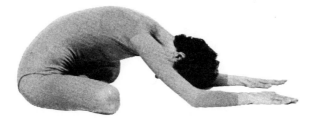

Relaxercises (2)

Sit with the ankles crossed, hands resting on the knees. Execute each of the following movements four times:

1. Keeping the head totally relaxed and loose, roll it in a slow, circular motion.
2. Shrug the shoulders up and down (together or one at a time).
3. Tilt the head forward and back.
4. Rotate the shoulders in a slow, backward motion (together or one at a time).

Repeat as many times as you wish.

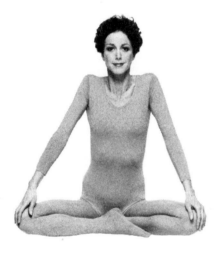 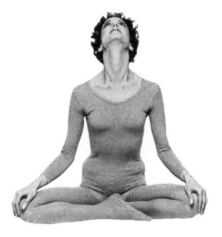

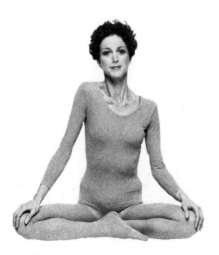 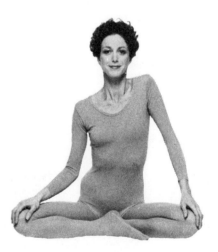

Relaxercises (3)

Sit on your heels. Round your body so that your head and arms rest on the floor. Maintain this position for about one minute. Inhale deeply and uncurl the body slowly. Repeat as many times as you wish.

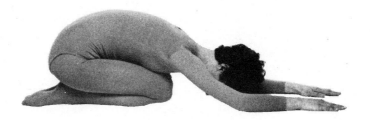

Relaxercises (4)

Lie on your back, draw your knees to your chest. Close your eyes and concentrate on your deep breathing (inhale through the nose, exhale through the mouth). If your neck is at all tense or tired, roll your head from side to side in a slow, relaxed manner.

This movement is particularly effective for relieving back strain and fatigue.

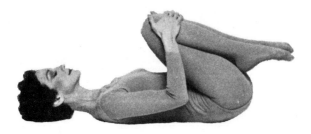

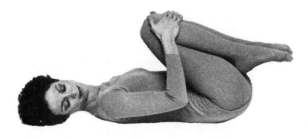

Glossary of Terms

The following defines the dance-oriented terms that I have used in the course of this book:

CONTRACTION: A tightening of the muscles.

EXTENSION: Stretching or straightening the leg at any angle to the body.

FLEX: This refers to the position of your feet. When you flex your foot, the toes are pulled back toward your leg and the heel is pressed forward. Flexing is the opposite of pointing, which is when the toes are pushed forward and downward, thus elongating the line of the leg.

GRIP: To tighten or contract (i.e., the buttocks or abdominals).

PLIÉ: In ballet, the bending of the knees. A grand plié designates a deep bend with a raising of the heels off the floor. The demi-plié (see Limber-Up ※7) is the bending of the knees as far as they can go without lifting the heels off the floor.

TURN-OUT: A basic position in which the legs are turned outward from the hip sockets.

UNCURLING: The slow, gradual process of straightening the body (vertebra by vertebra) after the back has been rounded. The movement should begin with the lower spine.